Living Life To Its Fullest™

Living
Life
To Its
Fullest™

Stories of Occupational Therapy

Edited by Ashley Hofmann and Molly Strzelecki
Foreword by Rebecca Austill-Clausen, MS, OTR/L, FAOTA

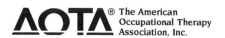

AOTA Centennial Vision
We envision that occupational therapy is a powerful, widely recognized, science-driven, and evidence-based profession with a globally connected and diverse workforce meeting society's occupational needs.

Mission Statement
The American Occupational Therapy Association advances the quality, availability, use, and support of occupational therapy through standard-setting, advocacy, education, and research on behalf of its members and the public.

AOTA Staff
Frederick P. Somers, *Executive Director*
Christopher M. Bluhm, *Chief Operating Officer*

Chris Davis, *Director, AOTA Press*
Victoria Davis, *Editorial Assistant*

Beth Ledford, *Director, Marketing*
Emily Zhang, *Technology Marketing Specialist*
Jennifer Folden, *Marketing Specialist*

American Occupational Therapy Association, Inc.
4720 Montgomery Lane
PO Box 31220
Bethesda, MD 20814
Phone: 301-652-AOTA (2682)
TDD: 800-377-8555
Fax: 301-652-7711
www.aota.org
To order: 1-877-404-AOTA or store.aota.org

Disclaimers
This publication is designed to provide accurate and authoritative information in regard to the subject matter covered. It is sold or distributed with the understanding that the publisher is not engaged in rendering legal, accounting, or other professional service. If legal advice or other expert assistance is required, the services of a competent professional person should be sought.
—*From the Declaration of Principles jointly adopted by the American Bar Association and a Committee of Publishers and Associations*

It is the objective of the American Occupational Therapy Association to be a forum for free expression and interchange of ideas. The opinions expressed by the contributors to this work are their own and not necessarily those of the American Occupational Therapy Association.

ISBN-13: 978-1-56900-294-0

Library of Congress Control Number: 2010922161

Cover Design by Mike Melletz
Composition by Auburn Associates, Inc., Baltimore, MD
Printed by Automated Graphic Systems, Inc., White Plains, MD

Contents

Part VII. New Pathways 167

Contributors

Beth Ching, MEd, OTR/L
Assistant Professor, Academic Fieldwork Coordinator, Level I
Samuel Merritt University
Oakland, CA

Penelope Moyers Cleveland, EdD, OTR/L, BCMH, FAOTA
President, American Occupational Therapy Association
  (2007–2010)
Chairperson, Department of Occupational Therapy
University of Alabama at Birmingham

Katie Corby, OTS
San Jose State University
San Jose, CA

Chris Davis
Director, AOTA Press
American Occupational Therapy Association
Bethesda, MD

Ami Dholakia, OTR/L
Occupational Therapist
Genesis Rehab Services, Potomac Center
Arlington, VA

Rhoda P. Erhardt, MS, OTR/L, FAOTA
Consultant in Pediatric Occupational Therapy
Private Practice
Maplewood, MN

Brian Estipona, OTR/L
UCSF Medical Center
San Francisco, CA

Rita P. Fleming-Castaldy, PhD, OT/L, FAOTA
Assistant Professor
University of Scranton
Scranton, PA

Sara W. Folsom, MS, OTR/L
Occupational Therapist
Department of Physical Rehabilitation and Sports Medicine
Franklin Memorial Hospital
Farmington, ME

Kristin Gulick, OTR/L, CHT
Occupational Therapist and Hand Therapist
Bend, OR

Sandy Hanebrink, OTR/L
South Carolina Branch Director
Touch the Future, Inc.
Chief Executive Officer
Wheeldogs, LLC
Anderson, SC

Jill S. Harris, PhD
Assistant Professor, Economics
California State University–San Bernadino

Ada Boone Hoerl, MA, COTA/L
OTA Program Coordinator and Assistant Professor
Sacramento City College
Sacramento, CA

Roger I. Ideishi, JD, OT/L
Associate Professor of Occupational Therapy
University of the Sciences in Philadelphia

Siobhan Kelly Ideishi, OT/L
Occupational Therapist
KenCrest Services
Philadelphia, PA

Leslie L. Jackson, MEd, OT, FAOTA
Project Coordinator
Easter Seals, Inc.
Chicago, IL

Heather Javaherian, OTD, OTR/L
Program Director OTD, Associate Professor
Loma Linda University
Loma Linda, CA

Alan Labovitz, OTR/L, CDA, CBIS
Occupational Therapist
Drucker Brain Injury Center, Moss Rehabilitation Hospital
Elkins Park, PA

Patricia Larkin-Upton, PT, MPT, MS, CWS
Clinical Specialist/Wound Master Clinician
Genesis Rehab Services
New Hampshire, MA

Patricia Mazur, MPT, BS
Physical Therapist
Home Based Primary Care
Veterans Administration
Daytona Beach, FL

Brenna Meixner, MOT, OTR/L
Occupational Therapist
Delmar, DE

Beverly Mulherin, MA, OTR/L
Occupational Therapy Consultant
Long Beach, CA

Rebecca D. Nesbitt, MS, OTR/L
Program Manager, Occupational Therapist
Genesis Rehabilitation at Aldergate
Charlotte, NC

Terry Olivas-De La O, COTA/L, ROH
Founder/President, Therapy Designs
Founder/Chief Executive Officer, Family Success by Design
Monrovia, CA

Charisma Quiambao-Fernandez, OTR/L
Staff Therapist
Genesis Rehab Services
Ormond Beach, FL

Shoshana Shamberg, MS, OTR/L
President
Abilities OT Services and Seminars, Inc.
Baltimore, MD

Carol Siebert, MA, OTR/L, FAOTA
Principal
The Home Remedy
Chapel Hill, NC

Barbara Smith, MS, OTR/L
Author and Lecturer
Hamilton, MA

Sam Smith
Hollywood, FL

Diana Steffen Steer, OT/L
Academic Coordinator,
CU/UAA Occupational Therapy Program
University of Alaska, Anchorage College of Health and
  Social Welfare

Jacqueline Thrash, OTR/L
Director of Rehabilitation and Occupational Therapist
Interface Rehab, Inc.
MSOT Student
San Jose State University
Glendale, CA

Meredith Umnus, PT
Physical Therapist
Genesis Rehab Services
Lake Geneva, WI

Marjorie Vogeley, MGA, OTR/L
President, Maryland Occupational Therapy Association
Columbia, MD

Rosa M. Walker, OTS
Sargent College of Boston University
Boston, MA

Rondalyn Whitney, MOT, OTR/L
Research Coordinator IV
Kennedy Krieger Institute
Baltimore, MD

Melissa Winkle, OTR/L
President
Dogwood Therapy Services, Inc.
Albuquerque, NM

Orian O. Zidow, OTS
University of the Sciences in Philadelphia
Philadelphia, PA

Foreword

I *love* occupational therapy and am delighted to write the foreword for this awe-inspiring book, filled with 35 remarkable stories. Each chapter highlights the joys, benefits, and purpose of occupational therapy in an exciting and entertaining manner.

As an occupational therapist for over 35 years, I am constantly challenged to define *occupational therapy*. I frequently request that people describe it in five words or less when I have lectured across the country about ways to market this wonderful profession. Students, educators, researchers, and practitioners typically sit for long moments of silence, then scribble furiously their own five-word definition. Each description is different and unique and attempts to capture the marvelous flavor of this multihued profession.

Still, it's important to have a single consistent brand—one common theme—when describing a profession. The purpose of a brand is to clearly identify a concept in ways that reflect all dimensions of the subject in an easily understood and succinct manner.

Occupational therapy is multifaceted. Occupational therapy practitioners work with children, adults, and elderly people. We treat people who have diseases or chronic and acute conditions, accident victims, and those impaired by psychological issues. Occupational therapy practitioners provide services in the community, people's homes, schools, clinics, hospitals, nursing homes, rehabilitation centers, psychiatric facilities, group homes, adult day care, hospice, and with the homeless. We work with adapted aquatics and therapeutic horseback riding. There are endless amounts of settings and clients that can benefit from occupational therapy. We are only restricted by the boundaries that we, as occupational therapy practitioners, place on ourselves regarding the location and services to provide. Occupational therapy is limitless, universal, and beneficial to all.

Occupational therapy is taught in community colleges, small- and large-sized universities, and most recently online. State and national associations proliferate as we share the professional exhilaration and scientific evidence behind this remarkable profession. International conferences are filled with excitement and camaraderie as we meet to discuss, share, promote, and communicate the joys of occupation.

So obviously, the task of branding occupational therapy is immense. How can five words capture the special flavor of this extraordinary profession?

To determine occupational therapy's new brand, interviews were held across the country for almost 1 year. I was delighted to receive a call from the marketing firm hired to listen to hundreds of practitioners, clients, educators, and researchers describe occupational therapy's uniqueness. Our in-depth discussions covered numerous thoughts and strategies on ways to capture the spirit of this amazing vocation.

As you ride in an elevator, how can you quickly describe occupational therapy before the doors open? Each occupational therapy practitioner can always describe their own unique position, but capturing the multitude of occupational therapy facets is challenging and tricky!

Yet, the essence of occupational therapy *has* been captured! We now have five words that describe the multidimensional profession of occupational therapy, and the stories in this book highlight the heart and soul of these five words!

Our mission, our purpose, our five-word occupational therapy brand is *Living Life To Its Fullest*™!

As occupational therapy practitioners, we are interested in all components of an individual's performance. We teach clients with physical, social, emotional, behavioral, or cognitive disabilities to live life to its fullest. Occupational therapy practitioners assist babies, children, and parents to live life to its fullest. We help clients in the community or recovering in hospitals to live life to its fullest. We educate occupational therapy students to live life to its fullest. Each setting, client, story, or person who comes in contact with occupational therapy is working on ways to live life to its fullest.

These five empowering words can be tailored for each occupational therapy practitioner's purpose. Our occupational therapy brand has a clear, common theme that encompasses occupational therapy service across all settings and across the world.

I remember one of the first times I described our new occupational therapy brand. I rode in a taxi to attend the American Occupational Therapy Association's (AOTA's) first Student Conclave in Chicago. The city was teeming with excitement, energy, and power. The taxi driver asked me why I had flown into the "Windy City" from my home in the Philadelphia suburbs. I explained I was attending an occupational therapy conference. Predictably, the taxi driver asked, "What is occupational therapy?"

Our new marketing brand had just recently been announced, so I took a deep breath and said, "Occupational therapy teaches people to live life to its fullest!"

Immediately the taxi driver smiled widely and proceeded to describe his version of living life to its fullest. We animatedly talked about the numerous venues of occupational therapy for the rest of the ride. I tipped the driver well as I left the taxi, thrilled that our new five-word occupational therapy brand had worked so effectively!

It is up to individual occupational therapy practitioners to personalize this brand for themselves and their practice. Using these five words in all conversations describing occupational therapy brings meaning, consistency, and clarity to our unique field.

The authors of the 35 stories inside have each personalized their occupational therapy–related experience of living life to its fullest. They share adventures of professional passion, love, advocacy, community integration, spirituality, roles, occupations, and purposeful and meaningful activities. Clients are restored and value returns to their lives. These stories will invigorate you and bring a knowing smile to your face as you read 35 remarkable highlights of occupational therapy and living life to its fullest.

AOTA has created many resources to assist occupational therapy practitioners in successfully using the occupational therapy brand. A poster, brochures, and wallet guide are all available on AOTA's Web site (http://www.aota.org/Brand.aspx). A new program called "Be a Champion for Occupational Therapy" encourages occupational therapy practitioners to promote and spread the word about occupational therapy by creatively and consistently using the brand's five-word phrase.

Living Life To Its Fullest: Stories of Occupational Therapy will inspire and excite you as you learn about 35 unique ways that occupational therapy has facilitated living life to its fullest. Enjoy the magic of occupational therapy as you read these stimulating and inspirational stories!

—**Rebecca Austill-Clausen, MS, OTR/L, FAOTA**
Austill's Rehabilitation Services, Inc.
Exton, PA

Preface

Before the American Occupational Therapy Association (AOTA) announced its new brand, the halls of AOTA's headquarters echoed with whispers surrounding what was cryptically referred to as "the sparkling words." We were dying to know what the new brand would be. We thought maybe we'd get a glimpse, a word, or a phrase here or there, but no. We would have to wait and be surprised along with attendees at the 2008 AOTA Annual Conference & Expo in Long Beach, California. Finally, AOTA President Penelope Moyers Cleveland unveiled occupational therapy's new brand, Occupational Therapy: Living Life To Its Fullest,™ during her presidential address (Moyers Cleveland, 2008).

After Conference, we kicked around ideas about how to make these very broad words *mean* something—to us and to those in the profession as well. One idea came bubbling to the top: Why not let practitioners and other people touched by occupational therapy illustrate what Living Life to Its Fullest means?

Living Life To Its Fullest: Stories of Occupational Therapy embodies that effort to articulate what occupational therapy is, how it contributes to helping individuals fully live their lives in ways that are meaningful, and how occupational therapy has helped practitioners develop and define their own lives and practices.

President Moyers Cleveland's address in which Living Life To Its Fullest first became synonymous with occupational therapy launches this book. Part I, "The OT in Me," is a collection of stories that show how the path to becoming an occupational therapy practitioner can almost seem predestined. Here, authors share the personal experiences that shaped their decisions to enter the profession or how they use their experiences to better meet their clients' needs. For instance, Beverly Mulherin's experience with occupational therapy as she recovered from a brain tumor inspired her to become an occupational therapist. Similarly, Rita Fleming-Castaldy's relationship with her brother and their experience of Friedreich's ataxia, a progressive neuromuscular disorder, convinced her to pursue a career in which purposeful activities and meaningful occupations could enhance the quality of life.

Part II, "Listen, Learn," highlights the art of teaching and supporting budding practitioners. Sara W. Folsom describes the inestimable value of having a good mentor as she seeks to become the best possible occupational therapist, while Rosa M. Walker shows that not all mentors who support one's occupational therapy career are necessarily occupational therapists. Ada Boone Hoerl gives us the professor's perspective as she slyly describes some of her tricks for engaging and teaching students—using buckets of dirt.

The heart of occupational therapy is, of course, its clients. In Part III, "Putting It All Together in Client Outcomes," nine authors share stories of clients who benefited in remarkable ways from occupational therapy such as Kristin Gulick's story of Israel, a client injured in a lumber mill accident, or Ami Dholakia's story of Ms. Martez, a young mother recovering from the removal of a brain tumor via a craniotomy. Roger I. Ideishi, Siobhan Kelly Ideishi, and Orian O. Zidow put AOTA's (2007) call for evidence-based practice from its *Centennial Vision* into action and describe how creating an inclusive preschool built on a solid, researched foundation can improve and change young lives. Heather Javaherian shows how it is possible—and important—to create meaning all the way to the end of life.

Some occupational therapy practitioners have had the unique experience of simultaneously being the occupational therapist *and* the client—in Part IV we call these brave practitioners "Insiders." Brenna Meixner and Jacqueline Thrash are each involved in a serious car accident, and they must call on their occupational therapy knowledge and skills as they begin down the road to recovery. Carol Siebert describes the balancing act of being an active, practicing occupational therapist while coping with the demands of Crohn's disease.

And every occupational therapy practitioner has his or her most memorable, most unforgettable client, such as Rondalyn Whitney's account of a remarkable husband–wife duo or Rhoda P. Erhardt's young client, Nathan, who learned to live and function with leukodystrophy. These stories and others appear in Part V, "Inspirational Clients."

Most occupational therapy practitioners already know how important their work is, but Part VI, "Client's View," tells the story of occupational therapy from the client's perspective, such as Jill S. Harris's story of her young son with Asperger's syndrome who delights in the activities of a sensory center or Chris Davis's insistence on seeing an occupational therapist after a stroke.

Finally, the stories in Part VII, "New Pathways," give a taste of the exciting, although perhaps uncommon, ways in which occupational therapy practitioners can expand their practice and promote their profession. For example, Leslie L. Jackson describes her wild ride of advocacy, from locally advocating for children and their families in schools to marching into the offices of U.S. senators. Barbara Smith shows how her various occupational roles of practitioner and caregiver led to work in the exciting field of hippotherapy, and Melissa Winkle demonstrates how dogs can be occupational therapy's new best friend.

Crystallizing exactly what it means to live fully is an impossible and arguably useless task. Instead, we present to you 37 writers and what they see as occupational therapy's ability to touch lives, allowing practitioners and clients alike to live life to its, well, you know....

Ashley M. Hofmann
Molly V. Strzelecki

References

American Occupational Therapy Association. (2007). AOTA's *Centennial Vision* and executive summary. *American Journal of Occupational Therapy, 61,* 613–614.

Moyers Cleveland, P. (2008). Be unreasonable. Knock on the big doors. Knock loudly! [Presidential Address]. *American Journal of Occupational Therapy, 62,* 737–742.

Part I

The OT in Me

CHAPTER 1

Be Unreasonable. Knock on the Big Doors. Knock Loudly!

Penelope Moyers Cleveland,
EdD, OTR/L, BCMH, FAOTA

Imagine the shock if the President of the American Occupational Therapy Association (AOTA) had been late for the presidential address at the AOTA Science and Exposition Conference. This year, I wanted to visually communicate my experience of the Centennial Vision *(AOTA, 2007) as illustrative of the metaphor of the "extraordinary journey," which I also used as the theme of my inaugural speech in 2007. Then, I was just starting the* Centennial Vision *travels; now, I am literally living this metaphor, because over this past year I have visited many members to describe our profession's vision. So what better way to demonstrate my journey than to have the audience believe I was stuck in the traffic of Los Angeles and that as a back-up plan, I was arriving by hot air balloon to the Conference in Long Beach barely in time for my presentation? There were pictures and sounds of me arriving in this manner. Once I "landed," which was made to sound like it was backstage, I appeared before the audience dressed in flight gear exclaiming that ballooning is an exciting way to travel.*

I know about balloon travel because when I was a new practitioner, I managed to arrange balloon trips across the Kentucky countryside for my clients with serious mental illness. Those trips were so exhilarating and magnificent! We all need such a source of vitality because here we are, less than a decade from celebrating our Centennial and achieving our Vision. And we have a lot of work to do!

Composer and filmmaker Robert Fritz (1984) said, "It's not what a vision is; it is what a vision does" (p. 122). Our extraordinary journey toward the *Centennial Vision* offers exciting opportunities for the profession of occupational therapy as long as we continue to travel on this journey together. Each of us—students, practitioners, educators, researchers, scientists, and retirees—has an important role to play in making sure that occupational therapy throughout the 21st century is a "powerful, widely recognized, science-driven, and evidence-based profession with a globally connected and diverse workforce" (AOTA, 2007). That is our *Vision*, our hope, and our goal. The *Vision* is what we are bringing into being, what we are inventing.

Knocking on the Big Doors

As we move forward, we will continue to be bold. We will continue to create and notice opportunities. We will be vigilant and resourceful in charting our next steps. We will be "knocking on the big doors" (Lemberg, 2007). (Paul Lemberg is the CEO of Axcelus, a business consulting firm and is executive director of the Cras Tibi Foundation, which raises funds and makes grants to organizations in developing countries.) These doors represent opportunities to meet the occupational needs of society and to realize the *Centennial Vision*. These doors will not open by themselves. Therefore, we will knock loudly. We will be—at times—unreasonable, because we cannot practice business as usual.

Knocking on these doors will take some of us out of our comfort zones. But we can learn something through clarifying moments that often are created when we try something new or set out to do what we have always been planning. I tend to have many more goals I want to accomplish than the time I actually have; therefore, I have to focus on the most important ways to balance my time in order to contribute to real and lasting change in the profession, in society, and in my personal life. Knocking on these doors to accomplish our Centennial goals requires us to step up *now* as leaders in our profession. If you are wondering, "Is she talking about me becoming a leader?" *Yes I am.* I am talking about each of us assuming this role. Our *Vision* will be what it does—to us and to our world.

Leaders I admire from the past opened many doors to change society and are a source of inspiration. Wilma West was a champion of our profession, as was one of our founders, Eleanor Clarke Slagle. Eleanor Roosevelt, during a dark time in our history, showed this country how to care for others. Heroes, however, are not simply those who deserve passive admiration. Rather than looking up to them, we would benefit more by looking *into* them; in other words, by emulating how they achieved such great goals (Chandler, 2001). Knocking on big doors is not easy, but if we each do our part, then many of these doors will open.

It is thrilling to learn that we are already knocking on and opening doors. AOTA's new partnership with Genesis Rehabilitation Services, employer of more than 5,000 licensed practitioners serving 150,000 clients a year in 21 states and the District of Columbia, is a prime example of the type of door to which I am referring. AOTA launched its new employer partnership program by combining the resources and talents of AOTA and this major employer to not only provide AOTA membership as an employee benefit but also enable educational and professional opportunities pertinent to the environment in which the Genesis practitioners work.

This is the first of many fruitful partnerships in which AOTA members ask their employers to fund their membership and to engage with AOTA in ensuring practice competence in this era of hyperchange, when knowledge is growing exponentially. How can we think about practicing, educating students, or conducting research without a strong professional organizational voice supporting us? Employers reap the benefit of your involvement in AOTA through your growth as a knowledgeable and competent leader in the profession.

We had an idea, saw an opportunity, stood up, knocked on the door—and now it has opened. Reaching out to employers is the kind of action that fuels our journey to the *Centennial Vision*.

Occupational Therapy on the Bypaths

Noted historian John Hope Franklin once said, "We must go beyond the textbooks, go out into the bypaths, and tell the world the glories of our journey." As our membership grows—partly because of employer partnerships—we are taking historian Franklin's words to heart and are taking the message of occupational therapy out into the bypaths. Not only the bypaths that lead to you our members, but also bypaths that lead to the larger world.

This year, AOTA leadership has held more than six town meetings and visited universities in many regions of the country. We have been to the University of Washington, Seton Hall University, Pittsburgh University, Tufts University, and Texas Women's University, to name a few. Leaders and staff also have presented the *Vision* during many state conferences and meetings and have described the related activities of AOTA. In these meetings, we create an opportunity to dialogue so that we know your aspirations for the profession of occupational therapy and what AOTA can do for you *today* to help you make your personal journey to the future.

Of course, the town meetings are important bypaths that lead directly to our members and to nonmembers, but what about bypaths that lead to the world outside occupational therapy? After all, following Franklin's advice to tell the world about our profession, or about "our glories," requires courage and leadership. Consider the example of our colleague Kerrie Ramsdell, an assistant professor of occupational therapy at Louisiana State University Health Sciences Center in New Orleans.

As we all know, Hurricane Katrina devastated much of New Orleans, but out of that disaster, Kerrie saw an opportunity, a door upon which to knock. She brought together charities, neighborhood groups, individual residents, and builders to integrate universal design into the rebuilding of the city. As a result of countless volunteer hours, many of the rebuilt homes have features that let their residents age in place.

Although Ramsdell's story is an excellent example of leadership and knocking on the right door at the right time, I have yet to describe the rest of the story! In 2006, Kerrie facilitated the initial meeting with me and the leaders from the National Association of Home Builders (NAHB), which then led both organizations to knock together on the door of AARP to create a significant collaboration. We are now all working together to promote livable communities that facilitate personal independence and engagement in civic and social life. A tangible outcome of this partnership is *The AARP Home Fit Guide* (2008), a booklet for consumers on home safety and livability. Occupational therapy is featured in this guide for its role in assessing the fit between the individual and his or her home environment.

Since last year's announcement of this partnership, a panel consisting of representatives from each of the three organizations has presented "Partners in Remodeling for Aging in Place" at several important conferences. In addition, I now serve on the Certified Aging in Place Specialist (CAPS) program Board of Governors, a part of the NAHB. A home builder, remodeler, or occupational therapy practitioner can earn the CAPS designation to market services as a specialist in this field. Occupational therapy thus has an inroad for actively facilitating teamwork between builders or remodelers and occupational therapy practitioners and for synchronizing this work with AOTA's own specialty certification in environmental modification. And remember, all of this was a result of one individual stepping up, taking a leadership role, and knocking on a door, thereby enabling AOTA to develop a synergy with two other powerful organizations.

Another example of being persistent in knocking on big doors is AOTA's cultivation of an additional partnership with AARP, this time also involving AAA. The CarFit program was born because we were unrelenting in wanting to show these partners the value of our perspective in helping seniors drive more safely. CarFit lets any driver, but especially seniors, meet with an occupational therapy practitioner and learn the various adjustments to the car that can be made to improve safety and driving ability. And now we have CarFit events across the country. We conducted CarFit during the AOTA Annual Conference & Expo in Long Beach and received media attention, which in turn helped educate the public about occupational therapy.

AOTA also is exploring a new path on the journey involving other potential partnerships. Mary Warren, associate professor at the University of Alabama at Birmingham, used her leadership skills in the occupational therapy specialty area of low vision to initially knock on the door of several relevant groups. Mary then pulled AOTA through the door with her. Now we are talking with the American Academy of Ophthalmology, the American Optometric Association, and the Association for Education and Rehabilitation of the Blind and Visually Impaired about a proposed model of comprehensive low vision rehabilitation services. We will continue working on how the organizations might support this model. Stay tuned for more information as this collaboration grows.

With our soldiers and other members of the armed services still facing danger overseas, AOTA believes it is important to promote the value of occupational therapy to the public in meeting the highly visible emerging needs of our veterans. We have been knocking on the doors of the Department of Veterans Affairs (VA) and the various military services to facilitate the use of occupational therapy on behalf of the injured. I have visited many sites that provide intervention and rehabilitation to returning warriors: Walter Reed Army Medical Center; Bethesda Naval Medical Center; and Intrepid National Armed Forces Rehabilitation Center at the Brooke Army Medical Center, Fort Sam Houston, San Antonio, Texas. At these centers as well as at the VA facilities, occupational therapy practitioners are doing incredible work with persons recovering from amputations, traumatic brain injury, burns, visual impairments, and mental health issues to enable these warriors to participate actively in society.

AOTA has opened the doors for members in other ways. We have held telephone "town meetings" with occupational therapy practitioners working in VA facilities across the country. We have learned about key concerns needing attention to support quality rehabilitation programming. Consequently, AOTA staff leaders began a discussion with the head of rehabilitation in the VA to address such issues as qualification standards, promotions, salaries, and continuing education.

And, we knocked on those really big doors on Capitol Hill. For the past 2 years, AOTA staff and members of the AOTA Board of Directors have been meeting with key members of Congress to be sure they recognize the utility and importance of occupational therapy to our veterans. And what do you think happened as the result of taking the time during our regular board meetings to knock on those doors? We obtained a chance to have witnesses testify before Congress!

On April 1, 2008, Carolyn Baum, past AOTA president, spoke before the important House Veterans Affairs Committee, informing them of the role of occupational therapy and research related to post-traumatic stress disorder and associated problems of living. Mary Warren also gave testimony on the low vision issues of veterans. We thank Dr. Baum and Professor Warren for graciously giving their time to deliver powerful and insightful testimonies.

We are continuing our emphasis on expanding our role in providing intervention for people with mental illness. This year, AOTA has been supporting mental health parity legislation, which has passed both houses of Congress. We are closer than ever before to having this legislation signed into law. AOTA also vocally and successfully opposed proposed regulations from the Centers for Medicare and Medicaid Services (CMS) that would have eliminated rehabilitation services in community mental health centers. This effort was accomplished through our continuing partnerships with the National Alliance for the Mentally Ill, Mental Health America, and the National Council for Community Behavioral Healthcare. In general, we are following AOTA's Long-Term Plan for Advancing Occupational Therapy in Mental Health Practice, which was submitted to the Representative Assembly (RA) for discussion here at Long Beach.

Leadership Development:
A Hallmark of the Moyers Cleveland Presidency

Whether we rebuild communities, promote independence for older adults, facilitate recovery from mental illness, or rehabilitate a wounded warrior, each of us has this ability to form an idea, seek an opportunity, knock on a door, and lead change. However, capability needs nurturing to develop into expert leadership in each of the six focus areas of our vision: mental health; children and youth; work and industry; rehabilitation, disability, and participation; productive aging; and health and wellness. We would have wasted time on our journey if our strategy had been to look for someone outside our profession to show us the way. We truly are professionals when we understand that no one is coming to do our work for us (Chandler, 2001). Instead, we need leaders within our profession to define where we are going and to find the byways to get to our goals.

As a hallmark of my presidency, I am focusing on leadership development. My belief is that each of us can be a leader, or that we each have the ability to craft what I like to call a "leadership story line." The story line is really a plan for becoming, being, and excelling as a leader. An innovative leadership story line contains three elements: values, ideas, and energy. A leader must be ready to articulate and reinforce the values of our profession. A leader must have ideas for how he or she might help achieve our *Centennial Vision*. And a leader must have a strategy to generate the energy to make those ideas a reality.

Values, ideas, and energy are within each of us; we use them every day when meeting the occupational needs of our clients, educating our students, and studying problems of occupational performance and participation. We now have to mobilize the elements of a leadership story line on behalf of our profession, and when we do so, clients will have access to high-quality and efficacious occupational therapy services.

Your leadership story might be to promote the value of occupational therapy each and every time you encounter a new client or his or her family—that is, reinforcing what you are bringing in terms of your knowledge, understanding of evidence, perspective, and skill—and how it differs from that of other professions.

Your strategy might be to make sure your colleagues in your hospital or agency or school really know and understand occupational therapy. Your leadership story outcome might be to never again have to vent, "My colleagues (or community leaders) don't know what I do," because in your leadership story, you have devised a plan to correct that lack of information. Or your leadership story might be grand, like that of Kerrie Ramsdell in New Orleans: to bring universal design—and occupational therapy—into a multifaceted dialogue about the rebirth of a city.

This is what Franklin means by going to the byways and extolling the glories of our journey. Lemberg (2007) tells us, "Extraordinary accomplishments begin with extraordinary ideas and are realized through extraordinary action" (p. 1). Are *you* ready to step up and lead through extraordinary action?

Many people ask me how I developed as a leader. My early career was in a system where female leadership was an exception, was not well understood, and, frankly, was not always welcomed. I had little experience because I was a fairly new practitioner, so I quickly sought out a mentor. But the important lesson I learned at this point on my career path was this: "No" is not an answer we should accept (Chandler, 2001).

I learned to be unreasonable and to turn no around and make it the question, "Have you been creative enough to achieve your objective?" If there was not enough funding for needed supplies from the budget, for instance, I learned to ask myself what was another way to obtain these supplies when told no. If our profession is to achieve the *Centennial Vision,* we need leaders for the journey who are full of unreasonableness and reject "no" as an answer.

To implement my leadership mission, we started this year with a Leadership Development Institute for our state association presidents. We also began, in conjunction with the American Occupational Therapy Foundation (AOTF), our second academic leadership program using the process of mentoring circles. This time, all the academic fellows are directors of either occupational therapy or occupational therapy assistant programs. The program focusing on state presidents—who are already on their own leadership journey—was designed to help the presidents motivate others in state associations, be effective communicators, deal with change, and recognize and nurture talent in others.

And AOTA is taking another step in promoting leadership. I am particularly excited about a new program called Coordinated, Online Opportunities for Leadership (C.O.O.L.), approved by the RA at this conference. C.O.O.L. will allow our members to submit their profiles online and be matched with potential leadership opportunities within the profession. It also will provide a source of candidates for the usual elected or appointed positions. We want to make working with AOTA a part of your leadership story line.

Did you know that occupational therapy students all over the country are writing their leadership story lines as well? The AOTA Student Conclave in Pittsburgh showed its participants the many doors that can expand the boundaries of their occupational therapy futures. Students received valuable tips for their next steps: how to prepare for fieldwork, land a first job, consider further education, and become an advocate for the profession. It was a great success, and I am proud to announce that we are holding our second annual Student Conclave in Chicago, November 14–16.

By leading today, these students become stronger leaders in the future. Thus, it is imperative that we develop their leadership skills and help them act on their values, cultivate ideas, and build energy.

Evidence-Based Practice

Success for our journey also depends on practicing competently, effectively, and efficiently. We are able to embrace science when working with clients because AOTA has been appraising and incorporating evidence in the revisions of our practice guidelines. The results of building evidence, along with the new challenge of defining and collecting outcomes data for occupational therapy, also are helping AOTA with policy and payment challenges, supporting our defense of the need for and importance of occupational therapy.

Still another way in which we are plotting our journey to the *Centennial Vision* is through the Research Advisory Panel, which was formed just last year. Research is fundamental to all the elements of the Vision: power, recognition, science and, of course, the underlying need for quality services. The panel, which is jointly supported by AOTA and AOTF, is making significant progress in revising our research priorities to better align with the main concerns of federal funding agencies and emerging social and technological issues. The group has already responded to requests for public comment on initiatives and strategic planning activities of federal agencies, highlighting issues of occupational performance as it relates to health and participation. By taking this step to coalesce the thinking of some of our best scientists, we are beginning to knock on the important federal doors of the National Institute on Disability and Rehabilitation Research and the National Institutes of Health to obtain a seat at the table, which is a key part of achieving our *Centennial Vision.* You can see that by being a member of AOTA and contributing to AOTF you are actively improving our research and leadership capacities.

I would be remiss if I did not mention the need for political leaders. Our political action committee, AOTPAC, is celebrating its 30th anniversary. Through the generosity of AOTA members, our PAC supports elected officials, regardless of party, who help the occupational therapy profession and its consumers, students, and scientists. The AOTA Board of Directors committed to 100% participation in AOTPAC fundraising efforts during 2008. I challenge other leadership groups within AOTA to encourage 100% of their members to donate. This is, after all, a major election year with potential for a great impact on the future of health care in this country. The word *powerful* in our vision depends on having a well-funded PAC compared with PACs of competing interests. We also need to be vigilant in making phone calls, sending e-mails, and initiating personal meetings with candidates and elected officials. By developing relationships in this way, we keep occupational therapy in the policy spotlight and advance our political agenda.

Telling the World About Occupational Therapy

Now is the time for each of you to take action and join our journey. I return to the words of John Hope Franklin. Remember, he said that "we must go beyond the textbooks, go out into the bypaths, and tell the world the glories of our journey." AOTA can help you by providing tools and by empowering you to lead, but we need each of you to go knock on the little and the big doors in your community and tell the world the glories of our journey to enhance occupational performance so that everyone can participate in daily life successfully.

- We can knock on the doors of our neighbors when we see them with an elderly parent in need. Occupational therapy has solutions that can help.

- We can knock on the doors of our communities by partnering with community health and service organizations to integrate occupational therapy into their range of services.

- We can knock on the doors of our universities to ensure that students who are in training to be health or service professionals in other fields know how we can help and support them as part of the team of service providers.

The age-old challenge that we face as we knock on these doors is, how do we define ourselves to the rest of the world? There are so many populations we serve and so many problems we solve. And who among us has not had to explain that the word *occupation* does not refer in a limited way to the activities of a person's job; it is a powerful term because the word reflects a person's *life*.

Fortunately, the *Centennial Vision* has moved us forward to aggressively address this lack of public knowledge that has haunted us over time. Using extensive research, including interviews with leaders across our profession, public opinion research, and AOTA member surveys and outreach, we have developed the sparkling words that we believe best define the essence of occupational therapy, both for us and for the public. These words are much more than a catchphrase or slogan. They are the foundation for a larger effort to "brand" the profession of occupational therapy. By building a brand identity, use of these words will enable us not only to knock on the big doors but also to make sure the doors open for us.

Ladies and gentlemen, let me unveil the next big step toward the *Centennial Vision: Occupational Therapy: Living Life to Its Fullest*™.

- When occupational therapy says the impossible is possible, we are helping people live life to its fullest.

- When occupational therapy works with a person with mental illness to set meaningful occupational goals thought to be beyond reach, we are helping that person live life to its fullest.

- When occupational therapy helps a wounded soldier learn to regain the balance and vision and perception to ride a bike again, we are helping him or her live life to its fullest.

- When occupational therapy inspires people to reach for the summit, no matter what, we are helping them live life to its fullest.

- When occupational therapy helps adults stay active in their own homes and communities, we are helping them live life to its fullest.

- When occupational therapy helps a child control negative behaviors and engage in positive socialization, we are helping him or her live life to its fullest.

We could and will go on with many other interpretations of our brand. Now we go forward with the message that living life and occupational therapy are inextricably intertwined. We will take these words—this brand, "living life to its fullest"—and use it in every aspect of AOTA's work.

We are developing tools to empower your daily practice and outreach efforts as we—together—knock on the big doors. I want to encourage practitioners to use the phrase when working with clients every day, when explaining the profession of occupational therapy to eager students, or when describing why our research ideas are so important to the health of our nation. We will include the phrase as part of our advocacy with policymakers. We will use the phrase in targeted advertising to increase our profile, giving us more opportunities to exercise the leadership to achieve the vision that all of you bring to this journey.

Yes, "living life to its fullest" is much more than a well-researched phrase. It is the tool that will help you make the *Centennial Vision* your own. Now is not the time for timidity. Now is the time for boldness. Now is the time to be unreasonable and to reject "no" as an answer. It is time to knock on a door you may not have had the courage to knock on in the past. It is time to lift your eyes up and disregard closed doors. It is time to live life as an occupational therapy practitioner, educator, or scientist to your fullest.

References

AARP. (2008). *The AARP home fit guide.* Retrieved September 12, 2008, from http://www.aota.org/DocumentVault/Documents/41878.aspx

American Occupational Therapy Association. (2007). AOTA's *Centennial Vision* and executive summary. *American Journal of Occupational Therapy, 61,* 613–614.

Chandler, S. (2001). *100 ways to motivate yourself* (rev. ed.). Franklin Lakes, NJ: Career Press.

Fritz, R. (1984). *Path of least resistance: Learning to become the creative force in your own life.* New York: Ballantine Books.

Lemberg, P. (2007). *Be unreasonable. The unconventional way to extraordinary business results.* New York: McGraw-Hill.

Note. Originally published 2008 in *American Journal of Occupational Therapy, 62,* 737–742. Copyright © 2008, by the American Occupational Therapy Association. Reprinted with permission.

CHAPTER 2

Independent, Active, Engaged, and Involved: Living Life To Its Fullest

Sandy Hanebrink, *OTR/L*

When I think about "Living Life To Its Fullest™" and occupational therapy, I must look at the roles occupational therapy has played in my life, and how occupational therapy has influenced my roles. I was first introduced to occupational therapy when my brother, Tommy, was recovering from neurosurgery. Although I did not fully understand occupational therapy at the time, I did know occupational therapy helped him figure out how to do whatever he wanted to do.

I later learned firsthand about occupational therapy after having a severe allergic reaction to an antibiotic resulting in transverse myelitis and quadriplegia. The occupational therapists, occupational therapy assistants, and occupational therapy students with whom I worked played an integral role in my recovery, became lifelong friends, and enabled me to do everything that I thought I could do and more.

As a patient, occupational therapists, physical therapists, speech–language pathologists, and recreation therapists began asking me to help motivate and work with patients they were having trouble getting to participate in rehabilitation activities. As we became friends, they valued my input. The therapists and students valued me and the role of people with disabilities. They knew the occupational therapy–disability partnership was the link to independence and living life to the fullest.

I began working as a peer counselor and attending in-services, asking questions and giving the user's perspective—as opposed to the perspective of the person treating a disabling condition—of durable medical equipment and assistive technology. Alongside my therapists, I became involved in fitness and recreation programs for people with disabilities. I soon became the assistant director of these programs. I also became a national champion wheelchair tennis player and Team USA Pan-American Games Wheelchair Basketball gold medalist. I helped start a wheelchair sports program for youth and took my first athlete to the national junior wheelchair games our first year. I was also involved with designing accessible playgrounds and advocating for access to recreation and the community as a whole. These peer-counseling opportunities, disabled sports events, and advocacy activities connected me to the world of vendors and the vast network within the disability community. Occupational therapy had helped me to access the world. It helped me to not only become independent but also to help others do the same. I was hooked on seeing how much I could accomplish and helping other people succeed and thus began my journey to become an occupational therapist.

I became disabled during the mid-1980s when health care and insurance allowed me to participate in rehabilitation services and get needed equipment. It was a great era and the beginning of innovation in technology, disabled sports, active involvement of people with disabilities, and disability rights. It was also a time of growth and expansion in services for the occupational therapy profession. I began to learn how to maneuver through government systems and programs, advocate, and—build vitally important networks. These were critical skills that I needed to become a successful occupational therapist and live my life to its fullest.

After state vocational rehabilitation department counselors and supervisors told me I could not be an occupational therapist because I was in a wheelchair, I began an 8-year battle in which I challenged the rehabilitation department systems in three different states to support my goal to attend college and become an occupational therapist. After several attempts at many organizational levels, I eventually knocked on the door of the Commissioner of the South Carolina Department of Vocational Rehabilitation and found success. I was finally on my way to occupational therapy school and a new set of challenges.

I thought I was joining a profession that helped people do whatever they wanted to do in life. However, to my surprise, I faced challenges from some instructors and occupational therapists who believed this—except when it came to being an occupational therapist. These individuals focused on what I could not do and not on how I could do it. I found this very frustrating—yet interesting—and was up for the challenge. I took each class as an opportunity to show the world that people with disabilities not only could be occupational therapists, but they could be the best occupational therapists. I wanted to prove that people with disabilities could do anything they wanted to in life and that occupational therapy practitioners could help make that happen. I found great support from many but continued to be challenged by others. These challenges helped me become stronger, more creative, and more persistent—skills that have been the foundation of success for me and my clients.

During occupational therapy school I stayed involved in disabled sports as an athlete and coach. I trained and competed in the Swimming World Championships in Malta and Atlanta Paralympic Games, winning silver and bronze medals, respectively. The athletes in my youth program also won the junior wheelchair sports championships as well as individual honors in track and field, swimming, archery, weight lifting, and table tennis. I also continued to grow as an advocate and served on the Mayor's Committee on Employment of People with Disabilities in Anderson, South Carolina, and helped expand the committee's role in supporting all areas related to disability. I increased my work helping people with disabilities and the people who serve them access needed services and supports. I became a resource for my fellow students and my faculty. I excelled in my curriculum and selected and set up my own fieldwork experiences that included working at a cutting-edge neuroresearch and rehabilitation center, a school for students with multiple disabilities and who were blind and/or deaf, and an internship at the American Occupational Therapy Association (AOTA) National Office. I learned from the best and began to truly appreciate the occupational therapy profession and AOTA not only for expanding my network of services and opportunities but also for how occupational therapy would help me and my clients develop the skills for the job of.

August was the anniversary of when I became disabled, and 2009 marked the year I had lived half my life as a person without a disability and half with a disability. Every year I have a Celebrate Life party on or around this date that usually includes a fund-raising event. The year 2009 was no exception. When I had my antibiotic reaction, no one thought I was going to live 22 more minutes much less 22 more years, and it was something to celebrate. I have been fortunate to have had many mentors and role models who have taught me and encouraged me to work hard for what I believe in, not only to dream but to have vision, to strive to take things to the next level, to lead by example, to facilitate and accept change, to respect everyone, to do the right thing, to play hard, and to have fun. I believe this is living life to the fullest. It is occupational therapy.

Since becoming disabled, throughout my education and my career, I have dedicated my life to helping others with disabilities, their families, and the individuals who serve them access funding, services, and supports to do whatever they want in life and achieve individual life goals. I not only work to help individuals with their specific needs but also advocate at every level from local to national to create change for all. I have helped write and advocate for new laws that improved opportunities for people with disabilities and occupational therapy. I have helped to develop new Social Security disability programs and policies and advocated on Capitol Hill and at the state and local levels.

My career and my life use my occupational therapy training and skills for success. I have been afforded and created many opportunities and am pleased to know that I have taken occupational therapy into the lives of many people and into professional and community arenas not traditionally known to occupational therapy, such as Social Security disability policy, leadership development training, and service dog training . As I have grown and experienced life, occupational therapy has gone with me.

I love to reflect on where I have been and where I want to go. My career in occupational therapy includes working in school systems, rehabilitation facilities, community programs, government service agencies, and private practice. I have helped parents learn to help their children thrive, taught children the skills needed to write and play, helped victims of trauma adjust, helped individuals get needed equipment to live independently, found needed technology for someone to work, fought to get someone out of a nursing home and back home, and helped someone die with dignity and peace. I have had the honor of seeing my clients go on to become healthy, educated, and employed; have families; and achieve greatness. I have helped others with disabilities become occupational therapists. I have presented and taught at colleges and universities across the country. I have written grants and obtained funding for individuals and organizations. I have served on local, state, and national boards and committees and have been an adviser on disability issues at the federal, state, and local levels. I have become a national expert and legal consultant on disability policies and laws. I have taught continuing education sessions and have written books and articles for AOTA, other occupational therapy events, and other health care professions. I have also written public policy and informational articles for the disability community. I have worked in major cities and rural communities. I have worked in individual homes, in schools, in corporate settings; trained and placed service dogs; and modified farm equipment. I have developed disabled sports and recreation programs, coached, and worked as an event official and classifier. I have modified and developed adaptive sports equipment. I have been an active member of my professional associations, held numerous offices, sat on committees, and served as chairperson of the Network of

Occupational Therapy Practitioners With Disabilities and Supporters since I was a student intern at AOTA.

I have found great joy in bringing occupational therapy to people with disabilities, as well as to all organizations and experiences in my life, and bringing people with disabilities and all organizations and experiences in my life to occupational therapy. It has been an honor to inspire people to see beyond disability, to help parents not to worry about their children but to dream about their futures and see those dreams come true, and to help people achieve independence and life goals. It is also an honor to help other occupational therapists live the profession and truly see the possibilities of all and help them achieve those possibilities, including becoming occupational therapy practitioners.

I believe we must not just talk about problems and oppression but act, present ideas, and work to facilitate change. And I dream of a world that is accessible to all and have a vision that AOTA and the occupational therapy profession will take the lead in making this happen. I believe occupational therapy has played a major role in developing my life and my life roles, and I am proud to be just one among many occupational therapy practitioners who do what I do and more. Occupational therapy is woven throughout all aspects of my life and has inspired many of the roles I have enjoyed. All of these experiences are a part of who I am and showcase how I live life to the fullest. Most important, they reflect how occupational therapy has helped me and my clients become independent, active, engaged, and involved.

Looking back, some of the things I cherish most include the independence I regained and the shocked smiles that I got from my doctors, therapists, friends, and family when I made it through that very first week and that I see each time I recover from a serious illness or do any of the things that no one thought possible. I cherish the memory of watching the parents' of the athletes on my disabled sports team hide behind sunglasses as tears of joy ran down their faces while they watched their children compete in a world that celebrated what they could do and not what they could not do. I value the smiles and energy these athletes gave me every time they came out to practice and compete. I get this emotional high when I watch a client achieve a simple task for the first time, and I remember the day when scratching my nose was living life to its fullest.

It is very difficult to put into words how much occupational therapy has affected my life. I am blessed to have had so many experiences and the opportunity to do the things that have meaning and value every day. I value occupational therapy. I value life. Knowing what it is like to experience traumatic illness, fight to live, regain independence, make new life choices, and live the life I want, and now help and influence others is a privilege. Occupational therapy has helped make this happen, allowing me to help others live life to its fullest and helping me live my own life to its fullest.

CHAPTER 3

Occupational Therapy: Reversing Adversity

Beverly Mulherin, *MA, OTR/L*

My story begins during my senior year of college. At 22 years of age, I was an active, independent college student, studying Social Ecology at the University of California, Irvine, working part-time, and earning good grades. But I was also experiencing many unexplainable problems, including severe headaches, occasional blackouts, and nausea. I was having frequent nightmares and mysterious fears. After seeing many physicians and undergoing numerous tests, a diagnosis was made: brain tumor.

The next months were filled with repeated surgeries and lengthy hospital stays. During that time, my once independent lifestyle drastically changed. For a few weeks, I was fed intravenously, and when I did start to eat solid foods I was unable to feed myself and needed to be fed by a nurse. I couldn't even roll over in bed! I had to call a nurse. My hearing and vision both became very poor. My stroke-like symptoms affected my right (dominant) side, and I became unable to write or walk. How was I going to resume my role as a college student? How would I succeed in life?

When I was in the hospital, I was introduced to both occupational and physical therapy. The occupational therapist would come to my bedside for my occupational therapy session. In those days, "crafts" were a really popular means of strengthening muscles and improving overall functioning. She provided me with a craft kit to keep in my room and work on when I felt like it. Unfortunately, I was too sick and my vision was too poor to do much with it. After 2 months in an acute-care hospital (long hospital stays were the rule at that time), I was sent to another hospital, which specialized in the next surgery I needed. Again I had occupational and physical therapy. By that time, I was beginning to feel better, although I still couldn't walk or write. The occupational therapist at my new hospital would come to my room, and we worked on activities to improve the function and strength of my right upper extremity. Finally, I was able to leave the hospital and go home to live with my parents. My doctor ordered outpatient physical therapy at a local hospital so I could learn to walk again.

One day, I was telling my physical therapist that I did not know *what* I could do with my life. I had lost my role of college student because I couldn't write or do other things that were necessary to be successful at college. She said, "I know what you need!" and sent me to the hospital's occupational therapy department. The department was wonderful. I did so many activities (including lots of crafts) designed to strengthen my right upper extremity, improve hand function, and increase bilateral use of upper extremities. I really loved occupational therapy and the occupational therapy staff and thought my occupational therapist was wonderful. I wanted to be just like her!

After several more months, I was again able to walk and write, although I was unable to accomplish either of these activities well. I went back to school to complete my education. Exactly one year had passed. Living on my own again was not easy. My balance was poor, and I frequently fell. Because I didn't write well, I found it difficult to carry out even ordinary school tasks such as note taking and writing term papers and tests. Because my vision was still not perfect and I was weak and not well coordinated, I was not able to drive an automobile. I felt and appeared disabled in every way.

But I kept trying. As I was finishing my undergraduate degree, a brilliant idea occurred to me. I thought how wonderful it would be to become an occupational therapist. I remembered that I had accomplished many things during my experience as a patient. I strengthened weak muscles and improved functional abilities, but I also increased my self-esteem. Occupational therapy provided me with the opportunity to be creative and to see a purposeful result to my efforts. It gave me confidence that returning to my previous valued role of college student was going to become a reality. I developed feelings of competence and usefulness and regained hope for the future. Because of the great experience I had in therapy, I felt like I wanted to spend the rest of my life helping others have the same experience. I was only a few weeks away from graduation; becoming an occupational therapist would require additional years of college—but it seemed worth the time and effort to me.

I needed to take prerequisites for the program before I even applied. I spent some time doing that, and then I applied for and was accepted into the master's degree program at the University of Southern California.

The occupational therapy program was difficult and very competitive, but I persevered, finishing my schooling and master's degree. I am so happy that I was able to receive such a great education! I have now been working as an occupational therapist since 1980. I have worked with so many people—from tiny premature babies to frail elderly individuals and everything in between! I have found my career to be most rewarding and fulfilling.

Because of my recovery and regaining functional abilities, I started to live quite independently. I had a very active life, which included driving all over and traveling to many foreign countries. One of my traveling adventures was the "Soviet–American Occupational Therapy Study Tour" in 1984. But I felt I needed a family of my own. I met a man who seemed just right for me, and we got married and started a family. My two daughters are beautiful! The oldest is now 20 years old and doing very well as a college student at the University of California–Berkeley. My youngest is just 12 years old and is a busy and active middle-school student.

My current position keeps me *very* busy. I am a self-employed consultant for adult day programs and many small group homes for individuals with developmental disabilities. At these many group homes and programs, I evaluate each client, looking especially at cognitive, social, and motor development; sensory processing; eating and swallowing abilities; and functional skills and then write treatment plans designed for direct caregivers to implement. I also make sure that each of the individuals served has everything needed (from an occupational therapy standpoint) such as adaptive feeding equipment, correct diet texture orders, hand splints and other positioning devices, and sensory equipment. I always look at the whole person and write a comprehensive treatment program, closely working with the staff to ensure the best possible therapeutic plan is developed and followed.

My experience has taught me that anything is possible. When a client increases his or her functional ability, I don't take credit for the improvement. It's all up to each individual. The occupational therapist doesn't make the client better. The *client* makes the client better. We just provide the right environment and tools that are needed. That's why the therapeutic relationship is so important in recovery. When in occupational therapy as a patient, I learned that the therapeutic relationship can influence and motivate a person to make positive changes in his or her life. It can really make a difference!

I appreciate all that happened to me when I was a young woman. I was introduced to a great career through what could have been a frightening and terrible experience. I have really lived life to its fullest thanks to occupational therapy!

CHAPTER 4

Honoring a Life of Loss, Resilience, and Meaning: Kevin

Rita Fleming-Castaldy,
PhD, OT/L, FAOTA

My brother, Kevin Michael Fleming, was born on October 14, 1954, and died December 8, 1989, from Friedreich's ataxia (FA). FA is a degenerative spinocerebellar disease characterized by progressive ataxia; dysarthia; and loss of proprioception, kinesthesia, and tactile discrimination due to degeneration of the cerebellum and posterior columns of the spinal cord. This autosomal recessive disorder also typically causes cardiomyopathy, myocardial fibrosis, and tachycardia, and eventually cardiac failure (Gillen, 2009). Because we were only 2 years apart in age, my older brother's lifelong struggle to live his life to the fullest with—and in spite of— a progressive neuromuscular disorder profoundly influenced the course of my own life. Because of Kevin, I found the field of occupational therapy. As a result of the disappointing, frustrating, and ineffective reductionist treatment my brother received from many of my professional peers, I became an educator. In recognition that even the most effective occupation-based interventions can be thwarted by systemic barriers, I have largely dedicated my professional research, publications, and presentations to the exploration, analysis, and confrontation of social policies that hinder the ability of people with disabilities to live self-directed, purposeful lives in environments that they choose (Cottrell, 2005a, 2007; Fleming-Castaldy, 2008, 2009).

In my previous writings (Cottrell, 1993, 1996, 2000, 2005b) and during many of my personal and professional interactions, I have observed that the gift of my life was Kevin. My brother's tenacious and unwavering quest to live life to its fullest until its untimely end taught me to live life with passion, integrity, and gratitude. These lessons were strengthened and continue to be sustained by the painful truth that my brother's life was full of loss, trauma, cruelty, and pain.

This story honors the complexity of Kevin's life and pays tribute to his achievement of a self-determined and meaningful life against overwhelming odds. My intimate knowledge of his life history guides my story. I describe Kevin's experiences with occupational pursuits and occupational therapy to facilitate an understanding of the relationship between these and living life to the fullest as exemplified by his life. But I undertake this task with much trepidation, because I know from the outset that my discussion will be grossly insufficient in conveying my brother's unique spirit. What follows is a very humble attempt to harness decades of memories and tie them together in a manner that will honor Kevin's life and the healing power of occupation, *when* it is person-centered and self-directed. First, some background.

When my brother was born, he seemed fine to our parents, and my birth followed 2 years later. They saw nothing unusual until the physical signs of FA began to emerge more clearly as my brother neared elementary school age. Popular (and uninformed) opinion at the time was that Kevin's odd posture was likely due to scoliosis. His awkward gait was attributed to his being pigeon-toed or bowlegged. Because our parents had scant financial resources and no medical knowledge, these explanations were accepted with the hope that my brother would outgrow the problems. When it became obvious that Kevin's physical abilities were continuing to regress, our parents sought a professional opinion at a publicly funded clinic.

After countless tests and endless hours fretting in waiting rooms, a diagnosis was confirmed. Unfortunately, the declared condition was not one that could be corrected with orthopedic shoes or a back brace as our parents had anticipated. Instead, they were told that Kevin had a genetic degenerative disease that would result in him becoming wheelchair bound by his teen years and probably dying before his 21st birthday. To add to the devastation of this verdict, the physicians observed that my parents should have known they were carriers of the gene that causes FA and not have had had any children. The fact that FA is a recessive trait that can skip multiple generations was never considered by the professionals or explained to my parents.

Burdened with unjust guilt and provided with no resources or support, our parents struggled to maintain some semblance of normalcy. They unequivocally rejected advice to place my brother in Willowbrook—the infamous Staten Island custodial care institution for persons with severe developmental, cognitive, and physical disabilities—and successfully kept him in our local parish school. Seeking counsel from their pastor, our parents were advised that Kevin was their cross to bear and that God justly and knowingly only gives you the amount of burden that you can bear. Armed solely with these empty platitudes and living in a society that viewed disability as a personal failure, our parents collapsed under the unfair weight of their heavy cross. Blaming themselves and perceiving no resolution to their grief, our parents coped as best they could. Our father sought solace each night after work in 2-quart bottles of beer, while my mother's angry isolation deepened into agitated depression. Battle lines were drawn that split the family. Our oldest brother, Dennis, could do nothing right by our father, while our mother only found fault in me. To keep the balance of power, our mother would defend Dennis, and our father would defend me. These confrontations were always loud and most often vicious. Each time, Kevin was caught in the crossfire, knowing that the angry rages were precipitated by our parents' helplessness in stemming the progression of his FA.

When the fury became unbearable, Kevin and I would retreat to hide under our back stoop. While we waited for the storm raging in our kitchen to abate, we would imagine how cool it would be if we could wiggle our noses like Samantha of *Bewitched* or blink our eyes like in *I Dream of Jeannie* to transport ourselves to a better place. Our haven's dirt floor provided the perfect surface for me to scratch, under Kevin's direction, intricate designs to tunnel out of our fenced yard. Alas, our escape efforts were as unsuccessful as the Hogan's Heroes we were emulating. Consequently, Kevin and I learned to seek refuge in books. Reading—Kevin, *The Hardy Boys*; me, *Nancy Drew*; both of us, Dickens and Twain—filled many hours. We also became rabid fans of the TV game shows *Jeopardy!* and *Concentration*, which nurtured a healthy sibling rivalry based on mental abilities.

This cognitive emphasis in our play was essential to our relationship because the physical destruction caused by FA made many activities impossible to share. So instead of playing ball, swimming, and bicycle riding, my brother and I played board games. Kevin's overshooting of the Monopoly squares and crooked Scrabble words were just part of the game to us. Equally normal were Kevin's calls for a redo of an erratic dice throw to get a more preferred outcome for his toss, his covert removal (when I went to the bathroom) of money stashed in his socks to be able to subsequently buy enough hotels to consistently bankrupt me, and his ability to accurately spell obscure words using Q or Z that resulted in many lost turns for me when the dictionary proved my adamant challenges of "that's not a word!" to be unfounded.

Despite Kevin's physical difficulties, we had spirited competitive games that lasted hours (and days for some Monopoly games) with much laughter (and some tears) as my brother teased me mercilessly. His ongoing jabs were always smart and often good-humored, but (as typical of siblings) there was the accompanying painful sting. Even though I rarely won, I loved these games, for I could see Kevin swell with pride as his *abilities*—his intelligence, cunning, and dry wit—shone. In those moments, my brother was whole.

Unfortunately, few people saw these nondisabled aspects of Kevin. Once my brother's FA became physically evident, he stopped being "Kevin" and became a poor unfortunate to be pitied. My brother's familial and social roles became solely defined as "the disabled child." His uniqueness as my incredibly smart and wickedly funny brother was lost to most of the adults in our lives. Kevin's sense of self was further desecrated by the cruelty of his peers. As a "cripple," bullying taunts, aggressive shoves, and derisive laughter dominated Kevin's schooldays. Gym classes and recess were particularly harsh as the teachers admonished my brother to try harder to accomplish impossible physical feats in front of a mocking audience. Some tormentors were particularly cruel. Often when Kevin fell they would kick his spilled books just out of his reach. As he crawled to pick them up and his hands were about to encircle them, they would kick the books again and again. This torture would continue until a kinder student or a teacher intervened.

Because our classes differed, I could not protect my brother while we were in school, but I could shelter him from bullies during our half-mile walk to and from school. As I helped Kevin up after he fell for the 10th time, I often wondered how to make things less painful for him. For years, my nightly prayers ended with a request to let me fall instead of Kevin because he was so thin. Having sought comfort in food, I was quite overweight at the time. Therefore—as I childishly rationalized in my prayers—I would have more cushioning and falling would hurt me much less. Of course, my naive appeal remained unanswered, and I eventually abandoned hope for divine intervention.

Our parents also tried their best to protect Kevin from the devastating effects of FA. Unfortunately, these efforts were equally futile. Our mother would consistently march into the principal's office demanding that Kevin's tormentors be punished. Reminded that there was a "more suitable" place (i.e., Willowbrook) for Kevin's "kind" and chastised to be grateful for our school's charity, our mother returned home filled with rage. Adding insult to injury, her angry visits to protect my brother meant the shame of "mama's boy" was added to the taunts.

In a desperate effort to make Kevin's legs stronger so that he would fall less, my father would strap my brother to an exercise bicycle and move his legs through countless cycles. I will never forget the stricken look of utter defeat in my father's eyes when he realized these efforts were completely useless.

The learned helplessness that pervaded our family grew exponentially with each trip to the public health clinics that our mother would drag my brother to (with me in tow) throughout our childhood. At the time, little was known about FA, so these visits most often focused on the documentation of Kevin's deteriorating physical capabilities. Because FA is rare, Kevin's examinations were typically performed with him semi-naked in front of an audience of physicians, residents, interns, and nurses. The thought that my shivering brother should be evaluated privately and with dignity never seemed to dawn on the crowd being enlightened who responded with "Ohs" and "Ahs" as the leading physiatrist traced Kevin's scoliotic spine. Only knowing nods of agreement accompanied the descriptions of how my brother's abnormal reflexes demonstrated neurological damage. *No one asked* how FA was affecting my brother's life.

Similarly, Kevin's rehabilitation highlighted his deficits. His physical therapy was dominated by endless walks between parallel bars as the therapists monitored the deterioration of his gait. Occupational therapy focused primarily on activities such as bean bag tossing to purportedly improve Kevin's eye–hand coordination. Although it was clearly obvious after my brother's first toss that he was *never* going to accurately hit the target, this reality was ignored by his therapists who urged him to "try harder." As children, we both knew this was just dumb, but no therapist ever veered from these established norms. The effect of these humiliating practices on my brother's sense of self was devastating. Years later, as an occupational therapy student, I wondered why no therapist ever considered teaching Kevin how to *do* things with his intact capabilities. Reading Gail and Jay Fidler's (1978/2005) classic work *Doing and Becoming: Purposeful Action and Self-Actualization,* I rued Kevin's misfortune of not having a therapist committed to these fundamental principles of occupational therapy.

With Kevin's "rehabilitation" reduced to periodic evaluations of his declining motor status, the cruelty at school escalating in proportion to his increasing ataxic symptoms, and his projected demise becoming more imminent, my brother's spirit was relentlessly beaten during his adolescent years. Yet Kevin persisted in his fight to stave off complete surrender to FA and its accompanying deep depression. Although he could no longer walk 100 feet without falling, he attended our local public high school, relishing the mental challenge of learning German and vehemently complaining about the uselessness of geometry. An avid fan of the space program, my brother never missed an Apollo space launch, mission transmission, or landing. These historic events provided an awe-inspiring diversion from the grim realities of Kevin's earthly existence (and one of the few excuses our parents would begrudgedly accept for an absence from school). Reading while listening to music continued to provide him hours of escape (along with a somewhat effective sound barrier to the never-ending kitchen wars). Nights made sleepless due to the pain of increasing spasticity were eased by listening to international radio broadcasts and writing requests for station postcards. Days became brighter when our mailbox was filled with postcards from all over the world that Kevin then used to festoon his bedroom walls according to continent of origin. Years later, when Kevin learned that American citizens who had received correspondence from Communist countries during the Nixon years had had their phones wiretapped for "national security," he very proudly recalled the numerous postcards from stations in Russia, the People's Republic of China, and North Korea that had adorned his Asian section.

Sadly, the mounting number of postcards cramming Kevin's wall space could not forestall the progression of FA. By his senior year of high school, Kevin could barely walk, but he refused to use a wheelchair for mobility because that would have meant the diagnosing physicians had "won." With the cooperation of teachers who valued my brother's intellect and spirit enough to waive their established attendance policies, Kevin graduated from high school. He did not attend the ceremony because it was in a stadium with multiple steps. Afterwards, a neighbor told us that when Kevin's name was called the entire senior class and faculty gave him a standing ovation. I will never forget my mother's tears as she angrily questioned where these applauders had been during the cruel taunts at school and Kevin's lonely days at home.

Having no post–high school plans beyond his impending death, Kevin's depression deepened and he became a recluse in his room. He still read voraciously and music continued to fill the air, but my brother's spirit was defeated. Fortunately, one day he developed a toothache that would not go away. As the pain became unbearable, Kevin recognized that he needed to leave the house to go to the dentist. Because his only remaining method of mobility was dragging himself across the floor, he also accepted the reality that he would need to use a wheelchair. My parents had no funds to purchase any mobility aids, so

I called every agency I could find in the phone book seeking to borrow one. After many dead ends, I was able to obtain a wheelchair from a pharmacy that had a contract with the Muscular Dystrophy Association (MDA). Thus began Kevin's association with MDA.

Prior to this development, I had worked as a hospital volunteer in an attempt to find something that would help Kevin. Through this experience, I was exposed to the possibility that rehabilitation can help persons with disabilities adapt and lead satisfying lives. This was quite a different perspective from the dehumanizing experiences of Kevin's childhood and led me to explore potential careers. When I learned about occupational therapy's emphasis on the use of purposeful activity and meaningful occupations to maximize a person's functioning and enhance quality of life, my life path became clear.

I began attending New York University (NYU) to obtain my occupational therapy degree and promptly had our family physician refer Kevin to an internationally known hospital for rehabilitation.[1]

The initial care my brother received seemed highly competent. He was given a custom wheelchair and scads of adaptive equipment to complete daily activities. As an occupational therapy student, I was impressed with these obviously skilled practitioners and their thoughtful interventions. However, it quickly became obvious that Kevin's greatest needs were not being met by the rehabilitation team. Most striking was the lack of interest in who Kevin was and what he wanted to achieve. As a 20-year-old living at home with no job or social network, Kevin clearly needed a complete occupational therapy evaluation. Sadly, the reductionist practices he experienced as a child prevailed, and his occupational therapy sessions largely focused on motor function, wheelchair mobility, and the self-care task of dressing. Although increasing strength and endurance were helpful to Kevin because his years of isolation had left him very deconditioned, sessions devoted to wheelchair mobility and dressing were physically difficult and extremely exhausting. Also, due to the nature of FA, the difficulty of these activities would only increase as his disease progressed. Dressing in the morning took a frustrating 2 hours to complete and left Kevin so fatigued that he could not hold a book to read or put a record on his turntable. This devastated my brother, for I had regaled him with images of occupational therapy making living with a disability more tolerable. To be so weary

---

[1]The remainder of this chapter is largely based on the prefaces I wrote for my dissertation (Fleming-Castaldy, 2008) and earlier texts (Cottrell, 1993, 2005b).

that you cannot enjoy life's pleasures is clearly sad; to have this fatigue brought on by an ill-conceived treatment plan was inexcusable.

Fortunately, my brother's assertive spirit reemerged, and he remedied this unproductive situation. He quickly (and loudly) refused to dress himself independently and threw out all adaptive equipment. This act of self-preservation was viewed by his therapists as a clear indication that my brother was a "difficult and unmotivated" client, and he was promptly discharged from rehabilitation services (he was allowed to attend the wheelchair clinic as needed). Not even upon discharge did any therapist ask Kevin about his values, interests, or goals. Luckily, I was continuing my occupational therapy studies and developing a strong appreciation for the holistic and therapeutic use of occupation. As I began to apply what I was learning to help maximize Kevin's abilities and compensate for his functional limitations (often using him as a guinea pig for course assignments), my brother began to envision a future beyond the four walls of his bedroom. He started attending MDA-sponsored group therapy and—for the first time in his life—Kevin left home for longer than a school day. Armed with a new point-and-click camera, my brother pictorially documented his inaugural week of freedom at an MDA summer "sleep away" camp. The pictures from that trip remain a treasure, because they show Kevin laughing with his fellow campers and their same-aged counselors with no stigmatizing barriers evident. These MDA experiences—combined with increasingly frequent forays with me into the world of live music—slowly but surely chipped away at my brother's self-imposed protective isolation. Consequently, he decided that while awaiting his demise, he should live more fully.

This resolution led to the decision that Kevin would become a student at NYU during my senior year so that I would be available to assist him with his transition to independent living. Predictably, many people tried to dissuade my brother from attending college because his FA was progressive. Family members, former teachers, college admission advisors, and rehabilitation professionals could not envision how Kevin could benefit from this experience (this was pre-ADA and his prospects for employment were nil). Kevin's resistance to accepting these imposed limitations was viewed by many as maladaptive and clear evidence of his denial of FA's terminal nature. Fortunately, one vocational counselor partnered with Kevin to achieve his goal of attending college to stimulate his mind, develop a social network, and live independently. My brother accomplished all these objectives with me serving as a novice occupational therapist and adapting his dorm and activities to meet his needs. Even with these adaptations, Kevin needed assistance with basic activities of daily living (if he was going to ever get to class on time), so he hired and trained fellow students to serve as his personal care assistants (PCA). With self-directed PCA, Kevin was able to complete his baccalaureate and graduate degrees. He attended concerts, dined in restaurants, partied during spring breaks, traveled to London and a number of cities throughout the United States, and lived independently in his own home. A self-determined life engaged in meaningful occupations replaced an existence of dependency and boredom.

Throughout most of these years, I often served as my brother's de facto therapist. However, to preserve our sibling relationship, we would periodically obtain physicians' referrals for occupational therapy to meet Kevin's needs as his FA progressed. Although I was always present when Kevin began working with a new therapist, I never mentioned that I also was an occupational therapy practitioner, for I was serving as a family member, not as a professional colleague. Invariably, each occupational therapist would competently assess Kevin's physical status, prescribe weighted utensils, and initiate a morning dressing program. Only one therapist ever asked my brother what he did for leisure, work, or meaningful occupation. This same therapist was the sole professional to question if there were any psychosocial needs that were not being met for Kevin and our family. Regrettably, this singularly gifted therapist did not stay in her position long because of a lack of administrative support for her holistic approaches.[2]

In response to these practices, Kevin would discontinue treatment after only a few sessions because they were "pointless." He again was labeled noncompliant, and I would resume my dual role of "sister–therapist." Often we would ask ourselves in frustration, what if I was not an occupational therapist? How could Kevin have learned to live life to its fullest with a physically incapacitating disability? My profession's literature was replete with holistic statements about the therapeutic use of occupation, yet my brother's decades of rehabilitation never ad-

---

[2]Years later I met this therapist at a conference and learned that she had been a student in her third month of fieldwork when she had first asked Kevin and I these critical questions. After completing her fieldwork, she had accepted a position at this facility hoping to effect changes that would enable client-centered practices. When her enthusiasm was crushed by the cynicism that surrounded her, she questioned if occupational therapy was the right profession for her. Fortunately, this therapist decided to change jobs rather than leave the field, and she reported that she eventually found a setting that supported the practice of occupational therapy in the manner she had sought to provide to my brother and our family.

dressed his valued roles of student, author, music lover, friend, and home maintainer. The realization that the core values of occupational therapy were rarely actualized in practice led me to become an educator. My mission was, and is, to help our profession's future practitioners understand that life can be (and should be) fully and uniquely lived by everyone, including people with degenerative diseases.

For many years, with the help of self-directed PCA, Kevin successfully achieved this aim. However, after a decade of independent living, the progression of his FA required more care than was allotted for home-based services. Since our family's financial resources were not sufficient to privately pay for PCA, my brother was forced to rely on public funding. Consequently, Kevin had to enter a nursing home to receive the PCA he needed. To ensure that this placement would not force him to reapply the shackles of his adolescent bedroom, Kevin and I interviewed the administrators of several leading facilities. The home we selected supported the maintenance of Kevin's personal control over his life, within the constraints of an institutional setting. We were able to recreate his beloved NYU dorm room, placing the map of the world on the ceiling over his bed and a poster of Jimi Hendrix burning his guitar over the toilet. A good friend (who had helped with all of the carpentry needed to make Kevin's series of apartments livable) continued his role as personal carpenter and custom made storage units that enabled every free space in Kevin's room to be filled with his favorite books, videos, and albums. My brother stayed up to watch Letterman after Carson, skipped the 7 a.m. breakfast, and frequently went to the local stores, restaurants, and clubs with me, our oldest brother, and his previous PCA employees who had become friends over the years. If a Springsteen, Stones, Mellencamp, or Billy Joel concert resulted in our return at 2 a.m., we just rang the bell and the nearest overnight-shift worker would let us in. While Kevin made the best of his life in this supportive environment, living in an institution still took away most of his choices and required the relinquishment of personal control over nearly all of his daily decisions. Consequently, the quality of my brother's life was greatly diminished.

During Kevin's 2 years living in a nursing home, we often questioned why the public funds paying for this institutional care were not available for home-based PCA. Because only a fraction of these funds would have been more than adequate to meet my brother's PCA needs, this institutional funding bias was particularly egregious. Consequently, we joined disability-rights organizations to advocate for legislative initiatives that would change PCA funding inequities. We also sought private funding for the development of home-based PCA alternatives. While these activities did provide Kevin with some hope, purpose, and meaning during his last years, the realization of his dream to return to his own home remained unfulfilled.

At the age of 35, my brother lost his fight with FA. However, the lessons he taught me about life and the questions his life raised about my chosen profession continue to influence me every day. Kevin's life deepened my understanding of the relationships among personal choice, control, occupation, and quality of life. As a result, I cannot (and do not strive to) separate my personal narrative from my professional self. I often use salient experiences I shared with Kevin as examples to underscore fundamental principles of occupational therapy to my students. My brother's life showed that how professionals work with people with disabilities can contribute to a denigrating existence of objectification as a diagnosis *or* to a self-determined life of meaning as a unique and autonomous human being. Based on the life I shared with my brother, the latter is the gift of occupational therapy, and one that we embraced years ago to empower Kevin to live his life to its fullest.

Dedication

This chapter is dedicated to my brother, Kevin Michael Fleming (1954–1989). Although Kevin could not win his battle with Friedreich's ataxia, his tenacious fight to live a self-determined life remains my inspiration.

References

Cottrell, R. (Ed.). (1993). *Psychosocial occupational therapy: Proactive approaches.* Rockville, MD: American Occupational Therapy Association.

Cottrell, R. P. (Ed.). (1996). *Perspectives on purposeful activity: Foundation and future of occupational therapy.* Bethesda, MD: American Occupational Therapy Association.

Cottrell, R. P. (Ed.). (2000). *Proactive approaches in psychosocial occupational therapy.* Thorofare, NJ: SLACK.

Cottrell, R. P. (2005a). The Olmstead decision: Landmark opportunity or platform for rhetoric? Our collective responsibility for full community participation. *American Journal of Occupational Therapy, 59,* 561–567.

Cottrell, R. P. (Ed.). (2005b). *Perspectives for occupation-based practice: Foundation and future of occupational therapy.* Bethesda, MD: AOTA Press.

Cottrell, R. P. (2007). The New Freedom Initiative: Transforming mental health care—Will OT be at the table? *Occupational Therapy in Mental Health, 23*(2), 1–24.

Fidler, G., & Fidler, J. (2005). Doing and becoming: Purposeful action and self-actualization. In R. P. Cottrell (Ed.), *Perspectives for occupation-based practice: Foundation and future of occupational therapy* (pp. 85–90). Bethesda, MD: AOTA Press. (Original work published 1978)

Fleming-Castaldy, R. (2008).*Consumer-directed personal care assistance and quality of life for persons with physical disabilities.* (Doctoral dissertation, New York University, 2008). *Dissertations and Theses Full-Text Database.* (Publication No. 3295337)

Fleming-Castaldy, R. (2009). *Disability, personal care assistance, and quality of life: A study of the relationships between consumer-direction and life satisfaction of people with disabilities who use home-based personal assistance.* Saarbrucken, Germany: VDM.

Gillen, G. (2009). Neurological system disorders. In R. P. Fleming-Castaldy (Ed.), *National occupational therapy certification review and study guide* (5th ed., pp. 147–174). Evanston, IL: TherapyEd.

CHAPTER 5

"This Is Not the Life I Had Planned"

Alan Labovitz, OTR/L, CDA, CBIS

We all have life experiences: good, bad, and indifferent. These experiences can be very connected to our professional behavior. We use our experiences to help guide us throughout life.

I myself have had a multitude of life experiences. I grew up, like many people, in a single-parent household. I moved around with my family, living in small towns and large cities. I lived in poor areas and more affluent parts of town. I remember not having much food in the refrigerator or the kinds of toys and gadgets some of my friends did. Living in a large city, I often got into trouble because of the people I was with and the choices I made. I had friends and acquaintances who wound up in jail or worse. I was often out of place with most of my peers because of our different lifestyles.

One morning 20 years ago, about 1 month before I sat for my occupational therapy certification boards, I got a phone call at my job. When the caller began asking me questions about my father, I was more curious than concerned. Then the caller said the words that remain clear in my memory to this day: "Your father has been in a serious auto accident, and you need to get here immediately." I'm not sure I heard much after that sentence, and my mind was like a bouncing ball during the 4-hour drive to the hospital.

My father had suffered a traumatic brain injury, multiple fractures, and numerous internal injuries. There were indications of a brainstem injury as well. But what I remember most were all the life support machines my father was attached to in the intensive care unit. I had so much to think about, but the doctor hit me with, "We need you to sign papers concerning potential removal of your father from life support." I told the doctor, "His mother is right here. She can sign." I was informed that as his only child, I was legally his immediate sole heir. Because he was not married at the time, I was the closest blood relative, so the decision was mine.

At 23 years of age, my world was crashing in. I recalled a conversation with classmates less than a year earlier. We were talking about how we all expected to care for our parents in our older years and how difficult it would be to do this just as we were really beginning our adult lives.

Before I knew it, there were hundreds of thousands of dollars in medical bills. Because I was the one in charge of my father's affairs, I had insurance and medical personnel calling me all day. Having to locate my father's important papers was another daunting task. I was still working full-time and trying to prepare for the occupational therapy board exams. Next, my grandfather got sick and entered the hospital. Suddenly, I found myself treating my patients for 8 hours per day and then going to see my grandfather and my father after work. One day I noticed that I had not even cried about my father and his situation. It would be a month and a half before this finally happened. I guess I believed that it was important to keep it together for my father and my family. I felt like the most stable person because my family was devastated and my father's friends were clueless about the severity of his injuries.

We got through the next 20 years. My father survived his injuries, but of course he was never the same. Time has moved fairly quickly, with many ups and downs. Everything that happened has helped make me a stronger person and, I believe, a better therapist. Understanding, empathy, and trust are important in a therapeutic relationship. Having varied and eclectic life experiences can enhance a person's awareness of the world around him. This insight helps to make us better people. But did I really need to go through this? The reality is that this is life, and it is what you make it.

I've often thought about how my life experiences are reflected in my professional life as an occupational therapist. Over the years, I have read literature concerning therapeutic use of self. The use of your own experiences is often an effective tool to deal with hardships and joyous events. Every day we use knowledge and experience to guide us in new tasks. Our medical model often dictates that we separate ourselves from our work. This model says we need to keep our relationships with patients and their families strictly professional. I'm not looking to be lifelong friends, but I do enjoy learning about my patients, their families, and their lives. Sharing something about myself and my life seems only natural.

Camaraderie exists among people with similar experiences. We can learn from each other, so I try to share my experiences whenever it can be of benefit. I've noted how patients' or their family members' expressions change if I begin a comment with "When my father had his injury." They become interested in how my father recovered and how I managed to deal with all of the stressors involved with a life-changing event like a catastrophic injury. Something that has struck me as interesting is how patients or family members' trust of the therapist becomes more evident when they know he or she has had a similar experience. Patients and their families are at one of the most vulnerable times in their lives with all types of medical and professional people providing input and direction. I've lost track of how many times I've heard people say, "I know" or "I understand" to these patients and their families. Quite often, patients and family members' reactions are, "How do you know? Have you gone through this?" So often we want to say what we feel is right, but we don't think about how it affects these individuals. But I can say that I know what they are going through—because I've been there. In fact, I'm still there.

Trust is also an important part of the treatment process. Trust and understanding are needed between the patient and his or her family members and the occupational therapist. We all have had good and bad experiences in our lives, but this does not necessarily make us any more capable of understanding someone else's pain or suffering. Many individuals have not had the same kinds of major tragedies or misfortunes in their lives as their clients. In these cases, the use of positive life experiences can be just as effective in gaining trust.

For example, while working in a psychiatry environment, I often had less-fortunate patients who viewed me as an educated, well-off person. They would tell me I had all these things they did not have, and that I did not understand them and their lives. To them we had nothing in common. I frequently would hang out on my unit after my treatment sessions were done and socialize with the patients, play cards, or do whatever was relaxing for them at that moment. If I talked about places we all had been or neighborhoods that were mutually familiar or if I made some street-slang reference, patients could see that I was a person like themselves and a bond would be established. When this bond is established, you can really affect someone's life. Once a patient asked me to attend his court hearing because he trusted that I would keep him safe. We are taught not to allow our patients into our personal lives or information, but we do this regularly in general conversation—not only with our patients but with many others with whom we have contact daily. It's only natural that we use this skill in our work setting as well as social interactions.

As a therapist for 20 years I have had the opportunity to supervise students, occupational therapy assistants, therapy aides, and new therapists. When supervising, I try to make this idea of therapeutic use of self clear and purposeful. Yes, grades, factual information, and skill sets are important to being a competent occupational therapist. But your social and communication skills and plain old common sense are equally important. Having the best grades or being the smartest occupational therapy practitioner does not necessarily make you the most competent person at your job. If you forget something, you can always look it up in a book or ask someone for the information, but inadequate personal or social skills affect your ability to interact with people in all types of settings.

I would not wish on anyone the bad things that have happened in my life, but I don't wish that I could live parts of my life over again. I have just tried to use these events and information to make sense of things. As a result, I have been able use my experience to mold my therapeutic style and skill set. I remember how I felt when I was the patient or family member. I want students and less-experienced staff to understand their own power of experience so they can be the most effective advocate and occupational therapy practitioner for patients and caregivers.

CHAPTER 6

OT Saved My Life: Surviving Domestic Violence

Terry Olivas-De La O, *COTA/L, ROH*

"Why do you want to become an occupational therapist? You don't need to go to college, just be with me!" was all I heard after being pushed down 12 flights of stairs and then dragged by my hair to my abuser's car. This was only the beginning of a year that began more than 20 years ago. Now I feel comfortable sharing why I did not finish my OTR degree, how proud I am to be a COTA, and how strongly I am committed to occupational therapy practitioners participating in every way with domestic violence services. As practitioners, researchers, educators, and students, we need to support those of us within our profession and whom we serve daily to understand how domestic violence affects so many who are hiding in undue shame and who are trying to find their occupation of living.

On that cold winter night more than 20 years ago, as I was being pulled from my apartment in my pajamas by an angry boyfriend and then left on a corner known as "hooker alley" in this area of California, I honestly believed that if I lived I would do everything in my power to become an OT, because this was my dream. When he returned to pick me up and bring me home, broken of body, heart, and soul, I felt I had nowhere to turn for help. The police had only warned him the last time he did this to me because they could not see my bruises. This time, when he was out of earshot, I called a classmate to come and get me; thank God for Linda, Bryan, and Roland, who were partially responsible for saving my life that night. Much later, I realized that I was also responsible, by asking them for help.

At that time there were few safe houses or hotlines (and I wasn't aware of any in my area). Many people, including law enforcement officials, blamed the victims or didn't see a need to provide special assistance. The domestic violence laws now in effect did not exist, so my abuser did not have to spend time in jail, even after I finally pressed charges. Without any options, I lived in fear with my friends for more than 3 months, hiding and praying not to be found. I had to make some difficult life changes. I dropped out of the occupational therapy program for 3 months and started work in a chemical plant, even when my dream since I was 11 years old had been to be an OT. How easily influenced I had been by "Joe." Each time I broke up with him he promised to be "better." Abusers make promises to their victims every day, and sadly we believe them for reasons only we understand. Somehow, I kept finding myself back in his and my deep, dark, secret cycle.

During this time I shared my "problem" with a professor to ensure that I would be able to continue in the program after my leave of absence. There was no domestic violence assistance in either the occupational therapy program or the university, and she simply encouraged me to continue in school. She could not understand my fear, and she and others asked me, "How could you let yourself get beat up?" (May I say here, it is my hope that none of my fellow occupational therapy colleagues say this to anyone at any time. Domestic abuse survivors already have enough guilt. We need you to offer assistance; do not give up on us, no matter how frustrated you are—we hear you, we just don't see any options.) Finally, I had to share with my parents that I was "not making it in school." I felt so ashamed that I could not give them the real reason. My concerned mom came to the university to speak with the dean of occupational therapy to see what we could be done to help me accomplish my dream, because she was not giving up. The dean's only comment was, "perhaps OT is not for Terry, maybe she should transfer to LACC [Los Angeles Community College] and become a COTA." I wondered, can't the dean tell there is something deeply wrong? Why was I prepared to help patients as an OT, but I couldn't help myself when I was in personal turmoil? How could this be changed, and more importantly, how could I change?

Unbeknownst to me, Joe had found out where I was working and got a job there. One day I found that my car's engine had been tampered with. When I went back to the building to find a ride, I encountered him in the hallway. He twisted my arm so hard that I later developed yet another bruise. Fortunately a coworker saw him, and I was called into the manager's office. She believed me and put him on suspension, which was all she could legally do at the time. However, as is common in abuse cases, her disciplinary action ultimately put me in more danger.

Two days later Joe was waiting for me outside my "safe haven." (I later learned from a police follow-up that he had been following me for months.) He said I was "going to pay" because I had humiliated him at work. I ran into the house, but he got inside too, yelling "you will never be anything in your life!" I thought I was alone when he pinned me against the refrigerator and began choking me, but a close friend and roommate rushed to my aid. As she hit him in the back with a bat, I escaped. That night, I made plans with my parents to return home, although I didn't share that I had been abused by Joe and instead put up a brave front. My brother and a friend arrived the next day with a trailer, and with many mixed feelings I returned home to be with my family and seek another career.

Two years before being accepted into the occupational therapy program, I had survived a horrific car accident and was told by the specialists that I could never be an OT due to my back injury. At that time, I was not about to quit because of an injury. Now, I again had to decide what my future would be. A year later, I found a rewarding path as an OTA. With the guidance of two outstanding occupational therapy professors at LACC, Karen Tabeck and Ellie Hilger, I was able to reignite my passion for this profession by learning the new skills and tools that I still use as a COTA.

In 2006, President George W. Bush signed the 2005 reauthorization of the Violence Against Women Act of 1994 (2005). A close friend read that Joe beat up another young woman so badly she almost died, and because of this law he ended up in prison.

I believe we can make a difference in domestic violence through educating, volunteering, and making occupational therapy a priority in the recovery of each person involved through the process of prevention, intervention, and recovery.

I strongly endorse occupational therapy being part of every domestic violence center, board, commission, and organization.

Survivors such as myself deserve the expertise and services of occupational therapy practitioners. I have the honor not only of assisting other survivors of domestic violence as a volunteer but also of dedicating my company and organization to the important work that is needed on behalf of all those whom we advocate for and serve every day.

My quest to be an occupational therapy practitioner saved my life by motivating me to continue my educational and professional journey. It inspired me to have strong occupational structure and to create justice for myself and others. I have also been honored to share my experience with other young Latina women. Recently, a former 13-year-old domestic violence client shared with me that she did not take her life after having heard my story and learning about occupational therapy tools. She is looking forward to attending college one day.

In closing, I would like to thank all OTAs and occupational therapy colleagues who strive to work in the field of domestic violence to make a difference on behalf of all women, men, and children who need our services each and every day.

Hugs from the heart.

Domestic Violence Statistics

- Abused women are 6 to 8 times more likely to use health care services than are nonabused women (Gazmararian et al., 2000).

- Thirty-seven percent of abused women first disclosed the abuse to their health care provider, which began their healing (Rodriguez, Bauer, McLoughlin, & Grumbach, 1999).

- The cost of domestic violence exceeds $4.1 billon per year in direct medical and mental health-care services (Pichta, 2004).

- Injuries resulting from intimate partner violence can force victims to take time off from work and lose wages, resulting in stress and even depression (World Health Organization [WHO], 2002).

- Rates of depression, suicide attempts, and substance abuse are higher in mothers who are domestic violence victims (WHO, 2002).

How OT Practitioners Can Help Survivors

- Be part of a safe house or group home to address communication, occupations, and self-empowerment. If necessary, start as a volunteer and find out how to become part of the staff or the board.

- Work with the site's domestic violence counselor, social worker, and psychologist on goal setting for clients. Be the client's advocate on all levels.

- Demonstrate occupational therapy's understanding of participation and occupational performance for self-empowerment of work, education, social participation, leisure, and all activities of daily living.

- Assist the survivor to address life skills for herself and her family (e.g., cooking together with her children, reading), and encourage participation by all those who live with her.

- Encourage survivors to get not just a "job" but to further their education to become self-sufficient.

- Reinforce leisure skills. Encourage survivors to take time outside of therapy to do fun things that are inexpensive but fulfilling: journaling, taking walks, doing embroidery, painting—help them find a passion!

- Help influence public policy and ensure that there is funding for occupational therapy to be an active part of domestic violence recovery.

- Donate items for safe homes: new undergarments, self-care items, and your time.

References

Gazmararian, J. A., Petersen, R., Spitz, A. M., Goodwin, M. M., Saltzman, L. E., & Marks, J. S. (2000). Violence and reproductive health: Current knowledge and future research directions. *Maternal and Child Health Journal, 4*(2), 79–84.

Pichta, S. B. (2004). Intimate partner of violence and physical health consequences: Policy and practice implications. *Journal of Interpersonal Violence, 19,* 1296–1323.

Rodriguez, M., Bauer, H., McLoughlin, E., & Grumbach, K. (1999). Screening and intervention for intimate partner abuse: Practice and attitudes of primary care physicians. *JAMA, 282,* 468–474.

Violence Against Women Act of 2005, Pub. L. 109-162.

World Health Organization. (2002). Violence by intimate partners. In *World report on violence and health* (pp. 87–122). Retrieved September 13, 2007, from http://www.who.int/violence_injury_prevention/violence/world_report/en/full_en.pdf

CHAPTER 7

It's Not Just Textbook—
It's My Heart

Katie Corby, *OTS*

There I was, sitting in a class called "disease and the human condition," when all of a sudden a wave of nausea hit me. I saw the room spinning, and it was all I could do to not burst into tears. Unbeknownst to my peers, I in fact, was not sick like I often times said I was, which was my common usual "reason" to excuse myself from lecture to walk to the bathroom feeling shaky and queasy. Studying all this medical information put my brain in overload and sent my poor nervous system into hyper-speed. These symptoms became were my constant companions my first year at San Jose State University's (SJSU's) occupational therapy program. I was suffering, but nobody knew to what depths. I was became familiar with these daily symptoms, and I knew the cause: the death of my beloved mother a few months previous to admission to the occupational therapy program. I was now 21, uncertain of who I was and dealing with overwhelming grief and insecurities that I could not understand. I was more confused than ever. I did not understand why I had chosen to come back to school after my mom passed.

All the medical facts, problems, and statistics from these first-semester occupational therapy courses were alive to me and freshly real. My mother suffered from a very rare bone marrow disease, amyloidosis—a disease that few people have of heard of. Put simply, *amyloidosis* is a disease in which your bone marrow overproduces an insoluble protein which then distributes and takes up residences in your major organs, causing them to fail.

In my my mother's case, distribution went primarily to her liver and then moved to her kidneys (which shut down renal function), and finally progressed to her heart, claiming her life. I watched my mother suffer from many of the conditions we talked about in my classes this first semester such as edema, congestive heart failure, kyphosis, acute renal failure, and falls. During my mother's illness, I saw firsthand many of the occupational therapy concepts we studied, such as adaptive equipment, energy conservation techniques, home modification recommendations, toileting assistance, transportation and community barriers, and various psychosocial issues.

I had lived inwith the reality of these concepts for the past decade of my life. This medical world was an all-too-familiar place, and the reminders of my mom's condition every day in class left me feeling overwhelmed and helpless. These occupational therapy classes seemed to be everything that I wanted to run away from.

I first heard about occupational therapy when I met some of my mom's therapists, and I decided that this was something that I could enjoy and do. My love of people and compassion for them overwhelmed my heart, and I knew that I wanted to be involved in a profession that restored dignity to those who were injured or suffering, fostered independence, and helped people live their best life. As I researched various therapeutic practices, occupational therapy was the profession that captured me. It enthralled me with its various domains and the limitless number of settings in which I could work. Occupational therapy was the perfect fit, and my mother encouraged me to the fullest degree to go away to college and become who I was destined to be, pursuing the occupational therapy program at SJSU. But she never saw me fulfill my dream.

After her passing—and in her honor—I decided to continue to pursue my dream, despite the physical and emotional toll it was taking on me. I suffered from strong anxiety and depression. However, although the occupational therapy program was the hardest thing that I have ever pursued, academically and emotionally, this program alone saved me from my anxious state and made me strong and autonomous.

Little by little, I noticed subtle changes creeping into my life. My transformation started during the first semester, when we students were asked to explore our own lives and identify what made our lives meaningful. Because I felt like my major role as caregiver to my mother had been taken away, I needed to gain an identity that was solely my own. Through the encouragement of my professors and through multiple classes, I was pushed to try new things and experience different cultures and events that I could have never foreseen. I volunteered in a women's shelter, worked for the American Cancer Society, attended senior water Tai Chi class, worked in a special education classroom, led my first groups in an elementary school, attended different support groups, participated in community outreach and health care promotion, worked in a mental health day program, worked in a pediatric clinic, got involved in student leadership, traveled all over the San Francisco Bay area for various projects and interviews, attended cultural festivals, and interviewed people with various diagnoses and from different cultures. It was through these combined events and reaching outside myself that I truly found myself.

As I progressed in the occupational therapy program, the opportunities got bigger. I realized that my own personal suffering and battles were not unique. By studying human functioning and disability, I became inspired by people who overcame all the odds. If so many people could conquer so much more than I was facing, I could get through this hardship.

In the occupational therapy program, I explored the various learning styles and found out what type of person I am: I lead with my heart. I also learned what other types of people are out there. By working through much conflict and many failures and pushing myself out of my comfort zone every single day, I am now an independent version of myself, open to embrace what life throws at me. But this independence resulted from sheer determination to achieve my long-term goal of graduating from school with my master's degree in occupational therapy. I draw daily from the inspiration of my mother, classmates, friends, and family, as well as the many people with disabilities with whom I have had the privilege of working. I see the barriers that some people have to conquer daily, and this humbles and inspires me. I have learned to seek joy every day in even the smallest occupations of my own life.

Despite the personal challenges that I've overcome to arrive at this place (graduating with my master's degree in May 2010), I feel as if I'm now a whole person looking at my life and learning to fulfill and be satisfied by my own occupations. Instead of letting my mother's long history of illness cripple me, I've found that it is often my greatest blessing, strength, and asset. When my classmates merely studied the facts and learned the statistics, I learned from a place in my heart. The subject of disability is not new to me, and I have had a lot of experience living with it. It also gives me my largest platform for relating to my clients. With empathy, I can relate to the everyday struggles, frustrations, and psychosocial issues that people with disabilities endure daily. Although their situation is hard, I hope to be real with them and give them hope.

In other words, the occupational therapy program saved me. I have a purpose: to turn disability into exponential possibilities.

CHAPTER 8

Creating a Life of Passion and Purpose

Shoshana Shamberg, *MS, OTR/L*

Thirty-one years ago, I was a single mother on welfare. I had dropped out of college to become a potter and start a production pottery business. After giving birth to my daughter, I suffered severe postpartum depression. I was exhausted beyond anything I had ever experienced, which impaired my memory and problem-solving skills and my drive to make it through the day. I could barely care for my newborn baby and had little energy for work, which felt physically and mentally overwhelming. The isolation of postpartum depression was devastating and felt endless, causing a sense of hopelessness and lack of motivation to see beyond my own pain and suffering. I also was forced to sell my pottery studio. Being a mother and potter at the same time was too overwhelming.

Prior to this point in my life, I had traveled around the world training with various artisans in a variety of cultures, including Native American, Asian, and Italian. I also had worked as a pottery and crafts teacher in various senior centers, early childhood daycare centers and schools, special education programs, camps, and a psychiatric activities program. These experiences led me to work at the Country Place, a psychiatric facility in Litchfield, Connecticut, where I was encouraged to continue my ceramics training and to eventually use creative arts to help those with mental disabilities as an art therapy aide. A short time later, Richard Beauvais and Phyllis Beauvais, therapists working at the Country Place, founded an innovative therapy center, Wellspring, in Bethlehem, Connecticut.

After the birth of my daughter and as the depression began to take over my life, the Beauvaises asked me to join them at Wellspring. They would provide the resources, space, and guidance to develop a ceramics therapy program if I would set up the ceramics studio and teach their patients the art of pottery. Under the guidance of their staff, I would use the pottery program to help facilitate the therapy goals of their patients.

In exchange, they would provide training, housing, meals, medical and therapy services for me, a small stipend, and a loving support system for my daughter and me. It was an offer I could not afford to refuse.

The pottery studio at Wellspring provided patients with a creative outlet for expressing themselves as well as a valuable sensory experience to help organize their nervous systems and enhance cognitive goals. The experience of teaching with such dedicated and creative therapists and helping such interesting people with psychiatric diagnoses was life transforming. At 25 years of age, I had found a professional slant for my pottery skills that provided unlimited challenge and enjoyment. I learned so much from everyone I worked with. I also realized that pottery was a tool I had used for many years in my own life to provide personal growth and healing from traumatic experiences and psychological wounds.

The positive feedback about the therapeutic pottery program from supervising therapists and the patients was extremely encouraging and energizing. The Beauvaises then encouraged me to continue my college education and look into the profession of occupational therapy. I had vaguely heard of the profession but had known only one woman who was an occupational therapist. She had greatly impressed me as a person and professional many years earlier, but I had never thought to ask exactly what she did. I was pretty ignorant of the details of the training and profession of occupational therapy. The Beauvaises let me know that with an occupational therapy degree, I could be paid more than I was as a teacher, and they would hire me to be part of their therapy staff once I became a licensed professional. I trusted my therapists, long-time friends, and employers—and decided to look into the possibility of pursuing occupational therapy.

I arranged an appointment with the head of the occupational therapy program at Quinnipiac College, Ruth Griffin. Quinnipiac College has an excellent occupational therapy program, and Dr. Griffin seemed intimidating to me—a very direct, seasoned, no-nonsense professional. During my first interview, she asked, "Why do you want to be an occupational therapist? And why do you want to come to the program at Quinnipiac?"

I naively and truthfully told her, "I really don't know. I'm just in your office because my friends—two therapists and my employers—suggested occupational therapy as a next step to developing my professional skills, and it seems like a good idea."

At that point she said, "This interview is over. I refuse to talk to you further until you do some research into the occupational therapy profession. You're wasting your time and mine right now. I'm going to give you some reading material to help. When you're finished, call me back for an interview if you still want to join us." She then handed me a huge, ominous-looking book, Willard and Spackman's "OT Bible." I almost fainted from the shock! She said, "Don't to bother returning until you have read this book completely and can intelligently answer my questions about occupational therapy. I'm expecting you to return the book—it's just a loan!"

I was devastated! For a college dropout who did not want to read any textbooks, this was a huge endeavor. Reluctantly, I took the book home and began to read it. I did not stop reading until I reached the last page. I stayed up all night and read every word like an addict. Everything I read resonated with my interests, skills, and life experiences. I quickly felt passionately committed to the idea of becoming an occupational therapist, but as a college dropout in three different programs, the last thing in the world I wanted to do was to return to college. However, I now had the knowledge and courage to talk to the intimidating Ruth Griffin. The second time I entered her office, I was able to answer her questions with smashing success! In fact I could not stop talking, and she let me go on and on and on. Upon her recommendation and with her guidance, I soon entered the program with access to grants and scholarships from the financial aid office as well as affordable, on-campus child care for my daughter.

The Beauvaises were happy for me and gave me their blessings when I left Wellspring to enter the occupational therapy program at Quinnipiac College at age 27. They wrote my reference letters and have been my support system ever since. I have returned to Wellspring over the years as a successful product of their mentorship, and have I provided professional training to the Wellspring staff. Healing myself has reaped tremendous benefits in a wonderful career as an occupational therapist spanning over 20 years so far, a master's degree in special education, five more children, and a wonderful husband of 28 years. Our children have chosen professions that show the influence of occupational therapy, education, and creative work. Our oldest daughter, who is now more than 30 years of age, has a master's degree in education, is an artist, and has worked at Wellspring in their elementary school, continuing the connection through generations. Our five other children are pursuing education and professions in the arts, psychology, and health care.

After 2 years at Quinnipiac, I had to transfer to Colorado State University (CSU) when my husband was accepted to graduate school in

Denver. At CSU, I completed my undergraduate degree, taking course work and fieldwork in combination with Quinnipiac College. I also had four more children while an occupational therapy student. I was a non-traditional student who was very blessed to have occupational therapy instructors and supervisors who believed in me and helped me complete my education.

Bobbie Steward, OTR/L, from Quinnipiac College, arranged all the details of my fieldwork, which was located far from her location in Connecticut, so I could move to Baltimore, Maryland, where my husband had gotten an excellent job. Bobbie helped me negotiate some very challenging circumstances that could have prevented me from finishing my degree. Elinora Gilfoyle at CSU negotiated my status as a nontraditional student who completed occupational therapy coursework and fieldwork over a period of 8½ years, while giving birth to four babies and raising five children (now six, I had my last child while in private practice) by my graduation in 1988 from CSU, with a bachelor of science in occupational therapy at the age of 36.

I put my own personal growth in pottery on hold for many decades while raising my "living, breathing, kvetching creations," my six wonderful children. However, crafts such as pottery, woodworking, and jewelry making always remained an integral part of my children's activities as well as my occupational therapy programs in pediatric school environments and handwriting programs in my private practice. I used crafts with my clients in private practice and the occupational therapy fieldwork students I supervised.

As an international speaker, I have promoted occupational therapy when traveling from Israel to Trinidad and throughout the United States, teaching others creative and innovative ways to use our occupational therapy skills and how to collaborate with other professionals for the benefit of people with disabilities.

When providing occupational therapy services as a public school therapist for high school students with severe disabilities, I encouraged them in their therapy and educational programs to develop a jewelry-making business, which served to teach literacy, math, writing, computer, and vocational skills. They raised income for themselves, the occupational therapy department, and their school, and they even donated a portion of their profits to charity. The creations they made were so professional looking a local boutique offered to sell them. The skills they learned making beautiful, unique jewelry carried over to all areas of their academic environment and were encouraged by teachers and other support staff. The school's principal and teachers were surprised at the students' independence, creativity, skill, and motivation as they witnessed them working and developing business skills.

As my own children grew older, more personal time for creative activities emerged. My connection with pottery and other crafts like jewelry making enabled me to engage in these activities for pleasure without the pressure of having to sell them to make a living.

When I became ill and disabled with Lyme disease in recent years, those activities provided crucial support for my own rehabilitation. They eventually helped me through my own disability when the pain and mental energy required just to perform basic activities of daily living was exhausting. Eventually, pain and muscle weakness, as well as mental and physical exhaustion, forced me to end my part-time school-system employment of 20 years.

Going on disability retirement was a devastating defeat. I felt imprisoned by a body that did not seem to want to heal, and the pain seemed like it would never go away. I fell down steps and had to walk with a cane due to muscle weakness, inflamed and loose joints, and visual–perceptual problems. I slept very little due to constantly adjusting my position to avoid muscle spasms. My home environment required adaptation for accessibility and safety, similar to the adaptations needed by my patients in my home modification consulting.

After 2 years of misdiagnoses of fibromyalgia and chronic fatigue syndrome combined with treatments and therapies that provided only momentary or limited relief, I finally was able to consult an infectious disease specialist who diagnosed my condition as possible Lyme disease. He immediately placed me on antibiotics, and I began alternative treatments like acupuncture and craniosacral therapy. Within a week, I began regaining muscle strength and balance, and within 4 weeks I had energy and increased range of motion and about 70% reduction in pain in my joints. It was a small miracle to finally find a doctor who listened and an effective treatment to begin the process of healing. Now, 3 years later, I am blessed to be healthy and energetic once again.

Once I felt a bit better after the antibiotic treatments, I had the energy and mental clarity to take charge of my health and wellness, which included physical therapy, occupational therapy, hand therapy, and massage therapy, as well as nutritional support and exercise in a warm-water pool, acupuncture, Tai Chi, yoga, pottery, bead and jewelry making, and environmental adaptations.

As a nationally recognized accessibility consultant, I never imagined how useful my knowledge about accessibility, home safety, building design, and construction for universal design would be in my own life. The barriers in my own home put me at risk for an accident and increasing stress. Handrails on both sides of all stairways were installed, which added to my safety and decreased falls. Due to severe inflammation in my hands and low muscle strength, all door knobs, faucet controls, and switches were adapted for easy manipulation. The height of my toilet seat and furniture was raised to make it easier and safer to get up and down. Full-spectrum lighting replaced the fluorescent lighting that hurt my eyes and caused strain and some visual distortion. I purchased a variety of kitchen and dressing aids to help me return to meaningful self-care activities with minimal discomfort.

Luckily, our home had been renovated previously using a design concept known as *visitability*, which includes adding minimal universal design features and accessibility on the main level of a home. Our home is almost 100 years old, and this renovation was an expensive and sometimes difficult process. Moving the washer and dryer to the main level eliminated two sets of stairs that I previously had to climb. The front-loading and stacked models minimized the need for bending and reaching. In the kitchen, the sink has levered faucet controls and storage cabinets have pull-out shelves. Skylights provide comforting lighting and sunlight. A ramped entrance enables visitors to wheel in, whether with a baby carriage, walker, or wheelchair. Our main-level bathroom is totally wheelchair accessible with side-transfer areas, pocket doors, a graded shower and bathroom floor with no partition, a hand held shower head, and a pedestal sink with levered handles. What a stress-free difference from our former home environment!

Occasionally, I must take antibiotics to control the recurring Lyme disease inflammation, but my immune system can now handle the stress, and my health quickly returns with few residual side effects. I have continued Tai Chi and yoga as a part of my daily living. Pottery has become my most treasured hobby, and I have made hundreds of beaded necklaces and earring sets for friends, relatives, and clients as gifts. Without the love of my family and friends, I could not have integrated all these parts of my life for personal and professional growth and healing.

Facing the reality that I will probably not be able to work with clients with severe physical disabilities again due to my physical limitations was traumatic at first. However, I adapted and found other ways to use my occupational therapy skills without the physical stress of my former job. My private practice, once part-time, is now full-time and is very flexible with minimal stress. Interesting ways to use my occupational therapy skills have emerged, such as consulting as an expert witness in litigation cases; assisting life care planners and trustees for people with disabilities; creating health and wellness programs for brain and body health; developing innovative sensory interventions to address visual–perceptual problems in populations with Lyme disease and autism while working with eye care specialists and educators; participating in professional advocacy; consulting to interior designers, architects, and builders; providing international training programs; mentoring and teaching on using the Internet; and consulting on the Americans With Disabilities Act (1990) to help employers and employees with disabilities stay on the job or return to work and adapt their work environments.

Sometimes, when living in the present moment, we do not realize how the traumatic challenges of our lives can create openings for personal and professional growth and healing. The present pain and suffering can seem an insurmountable obstacle, making it overwhelming to just face a day and function at a minimal level. However, sometimes we can achieve insight, often in retrospect, about how these challenges and traumas influence our own lives for positive growth, as well as provide openings and insights for others. As an occupational therapist, my challenges specifically gave me a deeper perspective on the challenges my clients face each day. I achieved a greater level of compassion and insight into how to assist them through the life changes, traumas, pain, and limitations caused by their disability and circumstances. As a result of my own disability I can more effectively help my clients and their caregivers manage the stress in their lives and find meaningful and healing modalities and daily activities to once again regain their roles, responsibilities, and enjoyment of life. I do not wish this journey on all therapists, but in retrospect, I can use my own circumstances to grow professionally and personally and not give in to despair and hopelessness but know that there is a light in the storm to help guide me through.

Reference

Americans With Disabilities Act of 1990, Pub. L. 101-336, 42 U.S.C. § 1232g.

Part II

Listen, Learn

CHAPTER 9

With Mentorship Comes Friendship and Professional Growth

Sara W. Folsom, *MS, OTR/L*

If you had asked me as an occupational therapy student what area I wanted to practice in, I would have told you, "anything but hand therapy." The complexity of it scared me. Today, I can say with complete confidence that I have found my niche in hand therapy, and it is all due to working with an occupational therapist and friend who has an infectious passion for what we do. It is my belief that when you find a mentor in the true sense of the word, you are experiencing good professional karma. Each day that I work with my mentor, Alice VanDerwerken, MS, OT/L, CHT, I become more confident and skilled at my job as a therapist. To have the opportunity to work with her is the single most important blessing of my career.

In March 2006, I graduated from occupational therapy school and immediately began applying for jobs (while continuing to study for my board certification exams). At the time, the hospital I currently work for, Franklin Memorial Hospital (FMH) in Farmington, Maine, did not have any open positions, but I sent my résumé and cover letter in anyway. FMH was the only place I had wanted to work since entering my master's program. I interviewed at several places and kept hitting dead ends. As luck would have it, I received a phone call about 3 weeks after sending in my résumé to FMH. The director of physical rehabilitation introduced herself and explained that she did not have a position open but that she would like to meet with me so that if a position did become available the interview process would be expedited.

Later that week, I sat with her and Alice, the therapist who is now my mentor, chatting about my experience and what I was looking for in my career as an occupational therapist. Alice was the occupational therapy supervisor and therefore would be responsible for guiding me through the process of becoming a new therapist. She sat in on the interview in order to get to know me better as a candidate. Three hours later, the director indicated she would be in touch if a position opened up, and I left with high hopes a job would soon become available. The meeting only solidified my feelings that FMH was where I wanted and needed to work. However, I would have to wait patiently for a position.

Three months later, I received a phone call from the director of physical rehabilitation letting me know one of the occupational therapists had given her notice. She called my references, and I was hired, beginning work as a new graduate at FMH in August. I took my board exams on a Friday and with excitement and apprehension started work on Monday. I was excited to finally be independent of books and the critique of professors and fieldwork supervisors, but apprehensive about the enormous amount of learning I still had to do to become what I felt was an efficient and competent therapist.

The day I went for my preemployment physical I was asked by the receptionist to go to the occupational therapy department to see Alice. I was welcomed with a basket of all the necessary goodies to study for my National Board for Certification in Occupational Therapy exam such as pens, pencils, highlighters, and sticky notes (as well as some jams and jellies personally made by my supervising occupational therapist). This was yet again an indication that I had found my home.

When I started at FMH, I worked in the school and pediatric outpatient settings and did some coverage in our acute care setting. After my 6-month probationary review, my director asked me if I wanted to start working with my supervisor covering our outpatient adult orthopedic and neurological patients. When I was in school, this was the area that most intimidated me. I reluctantly told my director that I wanted to accept this opportunity so I could professionally grow, but that I felt I needed to continue to build my pediatric skills and wasn't sure I could simultaneously do both. She took one look at me and said, "Sara, if you have Alice wanting to teach you, you need to take the opportunity." I could not argue. The skill and knowledge Alice possessed is unmatched when it comes to hand therapy. She has more than 25 years of experience and hand therapy certification.

In the spring of 2007, I began taking on a small adult orthopedic and neurologic caseload. Alice was there every step of the way and answered all my questions. We met weekly to discuss my caseload and review my documentation. Her insight into what I should be including in my evaluations and what I should consider when developing a plan of care fostered my independence and competence as a therapist. Occasionally, when I asked questions or she saw that I would be evaluating a patient with a diagnosis I had never treated, she would tell me to "look it up and get back to her." The way she taught me and coached me was in sync with my learning style in a way that is unmatched by any teacher or professor I have ever had. When I asked Alice clinical questions she would say, "Look it up and then we'll talk about it." This helped facilitate concrete application of the knowledge I was looking for. Alice would use current patients as case studies to further the application of this knowledge. I learn by seeing and doing, and Alice would always make sure I was in the trenches, doing and seeing the things I needed to. Her supportive nature made me feel that even though I did not know everything, that was okay, and I had the potential to some day possess at least a fraction of her skill and ability.

Today, Alice and I continue to formally meet every other week to discuss my caseload and anything else I need to review. I work side-by-side with her each day, and her passion for what we do is infectious. We treat patients in a way that I get to know her patients as if they are mine and vice versa. When one of us goes on vacation, she leaves her caseload in the other person's trustworthy hands. If I have a question during a treatment or evaluation, Alice is right there for me. If she has a patient she thinks I may learn from, she has me observe with her.

I believe that I received my job at the right time by being in the right place. I believe I received a mentor like Alice by having good karma. Not only have we worked together professionally and attended continuing education opportunities together, but I have been to her farm to pick strawberries, raspberries, and a few pumpkins. We even have a ritual of ordering burritos for lunch every Friday from a local burrito shop. Following a recent anterior cruciate ligament reconstruction (an injury from my second profession of skiing), Alice kept me well-fed with home-cooked meals and lent me several books to read to pass the time. She has always remained supportive of my professional and personal growth.

Alice has taught me not only the invaluable skills I need for a successful career but also the importance of mentoring. Mentoring is one of the best tools our profession has to promote its integrity and passion. Mentors like Alice ensure that occupational therapists like me continue to grow and devote themselves to the core values of occupational therapy. It is not enough to learn theory and practical skills in school and at conferences. We must observe those therapists who have grown with the profession and seen the changes occupational therapy has undergone to fully understand and appreciate the importance of mentoring future therapists. This is what mentoring has done for me. It has also allowed me to continuously take stock in my practice and ask myself each and every day, "How have I improved the lives of my patients and my profession today?"

CHAPTER 10

My Mentor, Mary

Rosa M. Walker, *OTS*

When I was 15 years of age, I cleaned house for our neighbor Mary to earn money for school clothes. I would vacuum the already spotless beige carpets, sweating and adolescently awkward as I maneuvered the vacuum cleaner around the gleaming wood tables, paintings, and sculptures from her travels in Africa.

Each week, she would give me a paper bag filled with glossy catalogs that she had already skimmed. What I remember most were the photos of luxurious cotton sheets. They were smooth, Egyptian, and of pale purple and blue hues. There were also silk pajamas that looked like they would slide through your hands like water, duvets, and pillows of all shapes and materials. I was fascinated by so many possibilities, so much fuss—who counted all those threads, anyway?—for the simple act of sleeping. This is what it must mean to be rich, I thought.

Mary was a regal, elderly lady, whom I never thought of as old. Her hair was always coiffed, her intellect sharp, and her attention tuned to what was happening around her. She asked me probing questions about current politics and what I wished to do with my life, and she urged me to borrow books from her extensive collection. I would, carefully easing off the dust jackets once home so as to not stain them with grimy hands.

She encouraged me to read and write deeply. And in the grace of her daily actions, she showed me how to *live* deeply, with courage and curiosity. Often, while drinking tea after I was finished working, she would tell me about her life. She spoke of being in a prisoner-of-war camp in the Philippines for 2 years during World War II; of the first time she ate a tree-fresh mango during her travels, relishing the juice running down her arms; and of the occupational therapist who encouraged her to do silver working when she was in the hospital with tuberculosis.

Most important, Mary offered firm encouragement of my dreams, slicing right through any hesitations I had about a new endeavor. Partly thanks to her support, I applied to Reed College in Portland,

Oregon, when others warned me against striving beyond the means of a student from a rural farming area attending a high school with only 100 students. Due in large part to her urging, after completing my undergraduate studies at Reed and earning a bachelor's degree in psychology, I splurged and used my savings to travel through Spain and Italy and volunteer for organic family farms.

On these farms, I did not sleep on sheets of Egyptian cotton. In Italy, I slept in a renovated truck, listening to the shifting sounds of the goats. In Switzerland, I slept in a stone hut, the air dense with cold. Everywhere, I slept intensely, with no need for expensive eye masks, silk pajamas, or sheets of high thread count, my dreaming mind sifting through days rich with new languages, places, and people.

If pressured to summarize in a few words what I gained through my travels, I would say a better comprehension of communication and community. I learned how to converse with people by gestures and body language, singsong Italian, and crucially, by listening to what lies beneath a person's words. Through exchanges of avocados and olives; recipes and meals; and frank talk about homesickness, hopes, and what it means to live a good life, with truck drivers, Peruvian immigrants, people at a meditation retreat, and family farmers, I gained an intense appreciation for how everyone, including me, creates community with each sincere interaction.

My experiences in Europe also remind me of why my chosen profession—occupational therapy—inspires me. In sharing work, daily life, and conversations with diverse people, I realized the capacity they have to change their daily realities, to exchange mediocre or "good enough" for better, to open the grip of their daily habits and insecurities, and to move toward a more satisfying and complete life.

While traveling, I was so caught up in what I was doing that my letters were sparse. I should have written more, especially to Mary. Two years later, and months deep into my occupational therapy master's-degree program at Sargent College in Boston, Massachusetts, my mother called to tell me that Mary was in hospice care due to chronic obstructive pulmonary disease with approximately 3 months left to live. Mary, this woman of precise lipstick, articulate opinions, and robust hugs was *dying*?

During one of my last visits, I sat in Mary's living room where she was intently watching the news coverage of the 2008 presidential election. Her skin seemed almost transparent, but her gaze was lucid. She looked so pleased to see me, and she reached out slowly to clear away the newspapers and books so I could sit beside her. She asked about my studies and what I thought about Boston. Had I visited the Harvard Museum of Natural History to see the glass flowers exhibit? "Exquisite," she remembered from decades back, recalling the details of the delicate glass flowers crafted with such finesse.

She talked in the poised, frank manner I remembered from childhood, speaking of how there was so much left in the world she had to learn—as she inhaled oxygen through thin plastic tubes—and then balancing that fierce yen with a comment about how grateful she was for what she had already done and experienced. She inhaled, savoring the crisp fall air coming through the window and the companionable moments with me, which were made brief by her increasing fatigue. Even in her final days she was a model of grace, a model of how to live with curiosity, courage, and an appreciation for immediate joys—such as an unexpected conversation with a friend and the melancholy aromas of fall air.

Mary, my mentor and dear friend, died in late November. Her spirit lives on within me in a persistent whisper that says, "Inhale, read, write, and live deeply." Largely thanks to Mary, "Live deeply," to me, means to learn—in that dopamine-rush of utter focus—new ideas, new dance steps, new countries, and so forth, and most important, to share that curiosity and knowledge with other people. What makes life satisfying to me are those moments when I connect with someone, whether a friend, an occupational therapy client, or a stranger, in that subtle, preverbal current of sudden understanding and humor.

As a future occupational therapist, I have some specific career goals: be involved in research concerning sleep quality and health, work with populations isolated by language and location, integrate alternative therapies into my practice, and constantly strive to better comprehend my clients. However, the most important contributions to my core values began 15 years ago when I met Mary. Since then my values have grown through my interactions with diverse and lovely people from many countries. These personal and professional values include creating community through genuine exchanges with other persons; to following my curiosity into new situations, places, and knowledge; and inspiring, questioning, and learning in equal measures.

CHAPTER 11

Lessons From a Bucket of Dirt

Ada Boone Hoerl, *MA, COTA/L*

Plant a seed, watch it grow. Start with dirt—various and sundry mixtures of peat and clay and rock and sand and gravel. Add light and water, some nurture to go with the nature, and before long, something new emerges. A simple task with complex results.

Gardening is one of my favorite occupations. Creating lush or colorful environments, watching flowers bloom or fruit grow, and feeling the sense of accomplishment and reward gardening brings me. There are many similarities between gardening and teaching, another cherished occupation that brings me some of my greatest joy. Combined, these two occupations help me live life to its fullest.

For me, students are like different types of seeds. Seeds need to go into soil that encourages their growth. In soil that is too dense or too compact, a seedling's tender roots cannot break through. If a student is in a class that is not suited for his or her educational background or interests, growth can be a struggle, and very little learning might occur. For some types of seeds, the planting depth is critical. If they are planted too deeply, the effort to break the surface of the soil may be beyond their means; if not planted deeply enough, roots have difficulty taking hold. Too much water can drown a seedling; too little can dry it out. Just like seeds, students have unique needs, and each responds differently to their environment and what they are given. One seedling always pops through the dirt, a large group follows, some emerge much later, and a few sadly don't make it in spite of all one's efforts. There is always that first student who quickly demonstrates ability ahead of others, the majority of students who follow, a few stragglers who finally "get it," and the occasional student who never does.

If students are seeds, ideas and concepts are the garden. Ideas energize me, while gardens inspire me. Students grow to understand and create ideas. I am energized and inspired by this process as well as the end results. Planning a lesson for occupational therapy students is like planning a section of a garden. What are we trying to achieve, and what do we need to do it? Are we growing vegetables and need lots of sun? Are we growing delicate flowers in summer heat and need lots of shade and water? Seeing the goal and orchestrating the outcome is a rewarding process that enriches my life.

From a bucket of dirt comes one of my favorite lessons. It is a lesson that has many layers and many interpretations: planting a bean seed. To plant a bean seed in fertile soil, water it, and watch it grow is a terrific thing to do. But there are so many other things this lesson can teach.

Reading about how the early practitioners of occupational therapy developed interventions so early in our profession helped me create the lesson. Grounded in occupation, using a task common to many, such as planting a simple seed, and requiring few supplies, they showed me how to create a purposeful activity that can be therapeutic, skill-enhancing, pleasurable for some, and educational for all.

The history of occupational therapy intrigues me. I am inspired by our founders, by their courage to be innovative and their leadership for change. I am always drawn to old pictures and writings that examine early treatment approaches. Hidden in the Dewey Decimal System card catalog, filmstrips, and purple mimeographs in the occupational therapy archives of the American Occupational Therapy Foundation's Wilma West Library, there must be a fabulous trove of treasures to explore. To spend a few days with that collection of artifacts would captivate me, fascinate me, and thrill me to no end.

When Ann Grady was president of the American Occupational Therapy Association (AOTA), a fabulous calendar was published, filled with pictures of our profession's past. My copy is a bit tattered now, but I love to show it to students and talk about occupational therapy history. Any chance I get to incorporate these types of pictures into a lecture, I do so eagerly. Blending discussions of history with the *Centennial Vision* (AOTA, 2007) triggers the crusader in me, ready to forge ahead into our profession's future with any who will follow in tow.

Like a little girl rapt in delight, feet swinging in excitement, I was on the edge of my seat during the 2009 Eleanor Clarke Slagle lecture presented by Kathleen Baker Schwartz (2009). Her words were inspiring, her stories were engaging, and her knowledge was vast. When it was done, I wanted to hear it a second time; once was not enough.

I recall a story describing the interaction between a restoration aide (i.e., an early occupational therapy practitioner before they were called "occupational therapists") and an injured World War I soldier. His "shell shock" (what we would now call "posttraumatic stress disorder") was no match for her innate ability to elicit engagement, stimulate volition, and help him find the entry to a pathway home. Paraphrased from memory, I can offer you this version:

Day after day the soldier would lie in bed, staring off into no-where. Finally one day, as he stared past the bedside table, the restoration aide placed a jar on the opposite table. Inside the jar were beans and a damp cloth. "Private Jones, I've started some bean plants for you. When they're bigger, you can plant them in the garden. They're here by your bed." And off she went to tend to her many other charges.

Not long after, the beans began to sprout. "Look, Private Jones! Your beans are sprouting!" At last, she had elicited a response. He turned his head to look, and then rolled in bed to see the beans better. He sat up to hold the jar and inspect the tiny plants in his hands. Regardless of where the beans were placed, Private Jones would seek them out and move toward them. He had reengaged with the world around him thanks to a restoration aide with clever methods and persistence in her therapeutic use of self. Rather than dismissing her patient as just another casualty, she sought an occupation that would stimulate him. Her determination to help her patient in a way unique to him is her therapeutic use of self.

Hands down, this one of my favorite stories. We can still use occupational therapy history as a tool to teach methods today. Interventions do not need to be complex; they need to be individualized. The power of the lesson is too strong to be allowed to entertain and inspire just me. So each semester, in my Introduction to Occupational Therapy class, my students plant beans. Of course, just as the restoration aide taught me, I don't tell the students what we're really doing, but I am as giddy as a schoolgirl in anticipation of the lessons to be learned! Lessons from a bucket of dirt.

After brief verbal instructions, I sit and speak no more. One by one the students come up. The rest of the group must watch each student complete the task and nothing else, attending only to the planting of the beans. No notes, no questions, no comments. I delight in watching the problem-solving, the adaptation, and the sensory reactions that occur without fail each and every time.

One after another, the planters file past the table set up with dirt and beans and cups until all have finished the task. The cups have drain holes, so each planter must problem-solve how to add dirt and sand without spilling it everywhere. Once they get the prescribed ratio of one-third sand and two-thirds dirt, they manage to coordinate the mess, the combination, and the instructions, some better than others. After watching almost 30 students, the last planters have figured out the most efficient and creative ways of putting soil, sand, and seed in a cup. The final step is to insert a wooden stick with the planter's name on it.

And really, they have no idea why they are doing this. They think they are planting beans—a logical deduction. They wonder if perhaps there is another lesson taking place. Yes, there is, but they don't immediately see it. But with probing questions, the real lesson begins to emerge.

I ask the students what it was like to watch the same task over and over. Some say it was interesting to watch how everyone had a different approach or how the methods changed over time. We talk about problem solving, modification, adaptation, peer-based learning in groups, and task attention. Others report that it was boring watching the same thing again and again. We talk about therapeutic use of self, body language, and the benefit an activity can have for a client, even if he or she has done it over and over and is tired of performing it.

I ask the students about the therapeutic benefits of the bean-planting task. They are able to generate a remarkable list in spite of being new to the profession. After they generate their initial list, we discuss the *Occupational Therapy Practice Framework: Domain and Process, 2nd edition* (AOTA, 2008) and talk about activity analysis, observation skills, and factual and objective reporting of behavior and actions.

I ask the students about the sensory aspects of gardening tasks. Some report a great disdain for touching any amount of dirt or sand and how they had trouble focusing afterward because all they wanted to do was wash their hands. To many observers, these reactions were quite obvious, while some masked their reactions rather well. Some students reported a love for the smell of dirt or running their fingers in the sand. We talk about sensory responses in adulthood and when to create sensory challenges, how to adapt tasks for those who avoid certain sensations, or when to forego a task altogether.

And really, they still have no idea why they planted beans. And I won't tell them yet. Class dismissed. As the week progresses, I tend the beans with light and water but never make any adjustments to the original placement of the beans. Most sprout and emerge within the first few days, and even those that were planted too deep almost always begin to peak out from the top of the soil by the time the next class meets.

The next class session begins with the tray of seedlings placed in the front of the room, and I deliberately run a few minutes behind schedule. Without fail, when I enter the room, there is a gathering of curious planters looking over their crop. This happens so predictably! Glee is the best way I can describe how I feel each time I see this. The lessons from the past are soon to be revealed.

With the tones and inflections of an old Southern storyteller sitting on the front porch in a rocker with a whittling stick and surrounded by the neighborhood children, I recite the story of the restoration aide and Private Jones and how a simple technique can have a powerful impact, reigniting a person's motivation and decision to reengage in daily life. Breathlessly hanging on to each word, the students listen. Every time, as expected, they suddenly become smarter right before my very eyes, understanding the power of well-selected interventions and discovering how to engage a client in meaningful occupations and activities. I can see it on their faces—they visibly change! They dab a few tears, sit a moment in silent reflection, and realize they've chosen the right career. They too want to emulate the founders who came before us and develop creative ideas to meet an individual's need.

We talk about maximizing engagement in occupations by "finding each person's bean." What is it going to take to get a client to roll over in bed as Private Jones did? What will motivate clients to put forth the effort to reengage in their daily lives? We talk about one's occupational history, about the importance of client-centered choice, and about selecting activities meaningful to an individual rather than as a rote reaction to, "Oh, I've seen this diagnosis before." We talk about occupation versus activity. We talk about culture, interests, and roles. We can talk about this all because of a bean.

For years now this has been a valued class activity, one that always renders me humble yet ecstatic, reflective yet anxious to begin anew. At the end of the course, the plants are in full bloom. The beans have grown, the students have grown. The stories have been told. I must store my supplies and bid the students adieu. Then comes the hard part: waiting for a new semester—a new planting season—so I can harvest the power of occupation and activity and once again extol the glories of the lessons from a bucket of dirt.

References

American Occupational Therapy Association. (2007). AOTA's *Centennial Vision* and executive summary. *American Journal of Occupational Therapy, 61,* 613–614.

American Occupational Therapy Association. (2008). Occupational therapy practice framework: Domain and process (2nd ed.). *American Journal of Occupational Therapy, 62,* 625–683.

Scwartz, K. B. (2009). Reclaiming our heritage: Connecting the founding vision to the *Centennial Vision* [Eleanor Clarke Slagle Lecture]. *American Journal of Occupational Therapy, 63,* 673–678.

Part III

Putting It All Together in Client Outcomes

CHAPTER **12**

At the End of the Day

Kristin Gulick, *OTR/L, CHT*

Israel came to the United States 15 years ago, leaving his wife, children, and parents behind in Mexico, coming here to work and earn money to send home to provide a better life for his loved ones. He returned home once or twice a year. He had completed the fifth grade in Mexico before going to work at various labor jobs. When he first came to the United States, his jobs included picking fruit in Florida, harvesting cotton in Georgia, and painting in New Jersey, but eventually he landed a job as a helper in a lumber mill. His favorite job was painting, because it was the easiest.

One day, 4 months after starting his job at the lumber mill, Israel's life changed forever. He was loading scraps of wood into a cart when another employee, who did not see him, pushed a piece of wood that knocked Israel into a large rotating blade. He remembers the intense pain and a bright light. He believes the light was with him to give him strength either for the life he would continue here or for the journey elsewhere if he should not survive this. He did survive. But, he would never be the same physically or emotionally. Israel was transported by air to a trauma center where they saved his life but not his right arm. The surgeons closed the amputation just below his right elbow.

The trauma center he was flown to was 3 hours by car from where he lived. He was told that he would have to relocate near the hospital to receive rehabilitation because the level of care needed was not available in his town. While Israel was processing the loss of his limb, he was also dealing with being uprooted and losing the support of the friends that he had made. His new home was a bedroom in a group home, and he shared a communal living area, kitchen, and bath with people he had never met. He was faced with reestablishing himself when he had not yet accepted the physical change in his body, his new sense of self, and how he believed others perceived him. Israel told me that he was taught that one was not whole without all of his or her body parts. He believed he was not a whole man anymore. He cringed at the questions. He shrank from the stares. He did not want help. He did not trust. His world was upside down, without direction, without hope, and without friends or family. All he saw was a man with one arm, and, in his mind, he was sure that this was all anyone else could see.

Israel chose a passive prosthesis that could be used either as a stabilizing assist or to carry very light objects that could be wedged into the preformed hand. Most important, it looked like a hand, and he hoped this prevented people from noticing his differences. Israel wanted to have increased grasp power and wrist rotation but would not consider any type of prosthesis that did not look like a hand. This ruled out the body-powered, cable-operated type of prosthesis that is most functional with a hook type of terminal device. His local prosthetist suggested a myoelectric prosthesis with a hand-type terminal device.

It was at this point that I met Israel. His insurance company approved the fabrication of a myoelectric prosthesis with an electric hand and wrist rotator along with therapy to train Israel how to use the device.

My first meeting with Israel culminated in the following general picture:

- *Orthopedic evaluation:* No concerns about range of motion, strength, sensation, scar, or posture. Patient would benefit from education about body mechanics and a home program for core stabilization and strengthening.

- *Prosthetic evaluation:* Patient requires continued controls training for function and confidence and training for activities of daily living (ADLs) and instrumental activities of daily living (IADLs), work, play, leisure, and social interaction. Patient will benefit from introduction to resources for persons with amputations.

- *Psychosocial situation:* Patient requires support for community reintegration. Patient will need to develop trust in provider to allow provider to motivate him to challenge his fears of failure. Patient is lacking self-esteem as well a sense of contribution and productivity. He appears to desire to engage but is challenged by developing a positive new self-perception and is struggling to overcome his fear of being viewed by others as different or limited. He would benefit from a strong positive internal dialogue that will help him deal with others reactions. Patient is receiving therapy with a psychologist.

Israel's occupational profile includes the need for improved prosthetic control to augment performance of ADLs and IADLs that will allow him to regain the confidence to engage in activities outside of his room and in the community. Restoring Israel's sense of independence and his ability to provide for others will significantly enhance his life.

An analysis of Israel's occupational performance reveals an inherently positive, fit, athletic, mechanically minded individual who, with some training and exposure, will quickly improve his motor skills, resulting in more consistent prosthetic operation and ultimately the confidence to participate in community activities. His fear of failure, public embarrassment, and standing out will require role playing in a supportive environment to practice difficult interactions.

Our first sessions were spent in the clinic completing an evaluation and developing rapport. Developing functional goals that are meaningful to the client with upper-limb amputation can require multiple sessions. I believe this is due to the complexity of recovery from losing a limb and how limb loss affects a person's life. All clients have some basic goals in common. The ability to identify goals that are meaningful to a specific client evolves with knowledge of the client, development of the client's trust, and the therapist's intuitive ability to help a person discover what is important to. We know when to wait, when to listen, when to push, when to ask the right question that elicits the answer the client has been searching for, when to advocate for them, when to teach the client to advocate for themselves, and when to help someone see beyond a bad moment to a bright future. These are our unique gifts.

For Israel, I came to recognize his desire to please, his drive to achieve, his need to be viewed as "normal" and not disabled, and the embarrassment and pain of his living situation. Taking these factors in to account, I developed a treatment plan. First, we set about training the muscle sites in his forearm that would be used to control his prosthesis. This task was positive for Israel because of his inherently good motor control and the computer-aided training that we used, which included visual rewards and competition. I quickly added therapeutic exercise that spoke to his sense of athleticism for general conditioning and postural improvement. I sensed that because we were just beginning to develop rapport I should start by working on the least personal ADLs (e.g., feeding) or IADLs before moving to personal hygiene. This would allow for development of trust. Prosthetic training includes learning skills both with and without the prosthesis and in all environments to prepare the client to be able to function in any situation.

I approached the idea of a home visit cautiously at first, although it would need to be done. I also knew that Israel had to become confident enough to use the prosthesis in public. It appeared that finances were tight for Israel. I also learned that he loved to go to a certain buffet-style restaurant, which would be the carrot on a stick that I needed.

Israel agreed to wear his new prosthesis out to the restaurant as long as I did not require him to use it. He was terrified that if he attempted to use it at this stage of learning control he might make a mistake and the prosthesis "would go crazy" and people would stare at him. I agreed to this arrangement and removed the battery so the prosthesis would not inadvertently activate. Sometimes we need to move in baby steps. We went to lunch, and when we sat down, Israel immediately placed his prosthetic limb under the table. As he approached the buffet line, I quietly suggested that he use the prosthetic hand to help support the tray. He did. When we returned to sit at the table, he rested the prosthetic limb on the table in a natural position and then looked around to see if anyone was looking at him. Everyone around us was engaged in their own conversations and meals. I sensed his relief. As we left the restaurant, he leaned close to me and said, "No one even noticed my arm." Baby step number one was successful.

We returned to the clinic to continue to work on improving control and confidence. We practiced that I was hoping that we could try in public the next day. At the end of the day I broached the possibility of a home visit. Israel was quick to respond with an embarrassed, "No, no. The people are no good there." I explained my reason for wanting to work in the home and mentioned that we could keep the visit limited to his room and avoid the common areas. I let him to go home and think about.

Our next visit involved more practice and improved control. As lunch approached, I suggested a quick walk to a deli while he wore the myoelectric prosthesis with the battery in and operational. He agreed with very little hesitation. We picked up our lunch without incident. On the one-block walk back to the clinic, I asked him to carry my bag in the prosthetic hand. He hesitantly agreed. As we approached the clinic door he was smiling. We entered the clinic, and he walked to the table, placed my lunch on it, and proceeded to unpack my lunch bimanually! Another successful step. At the end of the day he told me that he thought it would be okay if I came to his home for a quick visit. I had earned his trust.

Our home visit went well. It was short due to the meager living situation, but Israel had obviously been practicing using the prosthesis with any tasks possible in his room. Previously, I had introduced practicing handwriting with his left—now dominant—hand. He showed me the pages of practice that he did every evening at a very small desk in his room. I pictured him there alone at night devoted to improving his handwriting and felt a tug at my heartstrings for this man.

I had told Israel that we would fix lunch in the clinic at our next visit. When we arrived I told him that I would need him to go shopping with me to pick out the food. He would also practice some activities while in the store. He said that he would try, but that he was very nervous. I reassured him that I would be with him and help him with any situation that was uncomfortable. He was amazing. He opened those hard-to-open plastic bags in the produce section and loaded them with green peppers. He reached in to refrigerator cases to retrieve items. He reached high and low. He pushed the cart with both hands. Then came time for checkout and money handling. We stood in an aisle and Israel told me in a panicked voice that he was so nervous that he might drop the money in front of the clerk. Our practice in the aisle went perfectly. Then I told him, "Let's imagine that you do drop the money. What can you do? Most people would make a little joke of it or just apologize and pick it up. As humans we all make mistakes and most others understand mistakes. We all drop things." I asked him to remember an instance before his amputation when he might have dropped something in front of someone. None of us wants to appear clumsy or less than capable, so we make light of it and move on. With sweat on his brow he approached the checkout line. We chose a line with no one else in it to decrease the pressure. He handed the clerk the money, received the change, put his wallet away, lifted the bag into the cart, and pushed the cart out into the sun. The clerk never noticed that he had a prosthesis. I turned to look at Israel; we had matching smiles on our faces, and he said, "I get an A, don't I?"

Yes, Israel, you do get an A.

I now knew that he would use the skills he learned in the clinic out in public. If I had not taken the extra step of practicing these skills in the environments that Israel would need to use them in, I am not sure that he would have made that transition by himself. At the end of the day, it is outcomes like these that make me proud to be an occupational therapist.

CHAPTER 13

A Team for Kathryn

Meredith Umnus, *PT*

Kathryn was a lady 91 years of age whose wit and charm made it hard not to love her. She loved to playfully tease her therapists, and this made therapy fun for everyone. Kathryn had a very independent nature, taking pride in being able to care for herself and enjoying her apartment where she lived alone.

Kathryn was hospitalized for a heart condition and infection, which caused her to be weak and lose her independence. She came to our facility for rehabilitation with the intention of returning to her home relatively quickly. Unfortunately, she suffered another setback after only 4 days at our facility. During her therapy sessions, her therapists noted cognitive changes, as well as strength and coordination deficits. She had changes in her vision that made it difficult to read and use utensils for cooking. Kathryn also had difficulty expressing as well as understanding language. She returned to the hospital for evaluation, where it was determined she had a transient ischemic attack, which presents like a stroke, affecting one side of the body. Kathryn's symptoms primarily involved her right arm and language abilities.

Kathryn returned to our facility for rehabilitation with visual and memory deficits, right-arm weakness and incoordination, self-care deficits, and difficulty ambulating. To complicate matters, her knee was arthritic and sometimes unpredictable.

Kathryn worked diligently with speech therapy, occupational therapy, and physical therapy to regain all the skills needed to live on her own again. A physical therapist myself, I observed the occupational therapist use a wide variety of tasks to help Kathryn reach her goals. Therapeutic putty exercises were used to improve hand strength. Manipulating small objects such as placing pegs on a board or threading small beads on a string improved her fine motor coordination. Arm exercises with weights improved her large-muscle strength. All these tasks contributed to Kathryn's functional training with meal preparation, bathing, dressing, and leisure activities such as knitting.

Her three therapists (occupational therapy, physical therapy, and speech–language pathology) collaborated for treatment to work on activities that Kathryn would perform at home. This required coordinating skills from all three therapy areas. For example, cooking in the kitchen required problem solving and sequencing for recipes, fine motor coordination and upper-body strength for cutting and mixing foods, and safety and balance when walking in the kitchen and retrieving items. When therapists provide treatment this way, learning tasks becomes more concrete and readily applicable.

Kathryn also regained skills through many creative sessions combining mobility, balance, safety, strength, and problem-solving tasks that simulated "A Day in the Life of Kathryn." Kathryn baked cookies, made soup, knitted, walked in the kitchen, and planned parties with her therapists. All the while, Kathryn continued with her wit and sharp comebacks, keeping her therapists laughing by announcing, "I may be old, but I'm not dead!"

After 2 months, the time finally came for a home assessment, which made Kathryn very happy. Her occupational therapist and I performed the home assessment, resulting in recommendations to remove throw rugs in the kitchen and bathroom and to create a wider walkway from the living room to the kitchen to decrease Kathryn's risk for falls. The occupational therapist also recommended that Kathryn use a microwave for her cooking, given her visual deficits, due to a higher risk for injury when using the stove.

Recommendations were made to Kathryn and her daughter, and the two of them felt ready for her to return home. She was grateful to the friends she had made at our facility but anxious to return to her home. She had worked hard to achieve this goal. Before she left, she made sure to thank her therapists with hugs and tears of joy.

Kathryn's story is one of many that show how a team of therapists working together and a determined patient can make dreams come true.

CHAPTER 14

Preschool Inclusion and Community Participation

Roger I. Ideishi, *JD, OT/L;*
Siobhan Kelly Ideishi, *OT/L; and*
Orian O. Zidow, *OTS*

> *"Inclusion requires we ensure not only that everyone is treated fairly or equitably, but also that all individuals have the same opportunities to participate in the naturally occurring activities of society."*
> —American Occupational Therapy Association [AOTA], 2004, p. 668.

For the past 7 years, KenCrest and University of the Sciences in Philadelphia (USP) have collaborated to develop integrated therapeutic programs for children with developmental disabilities as well as typically developing children enrolled at an inclusive preschool. The integrated therapeutic programs include gardening, dance, and museum and aquarium community outreach programs.

KenCrest is the largest provider of community-based services to people of all ages with developmental disabilities in southeastern Pennsylvania. KenCrest's Children and Family Services division serves infants, toddlers, and preschoolers who have developmental, neurological, orthopedic, behavioral, and learning difficulties in inclusive preschool settings (KenCrest, 2009). The USP program in occupational therapy emphasizes active and experiential learning methods such as service learning, where a student's learning is paired with a community need for a mutually beneficial experience (Kramer et al., 2007). KenCrest and USP initiated a service learning partnership to meet KenCrest's need to develop inclusive therapeutic programming and USP's need to provide a rich and authentic learning experience for occupational therapy students.

Inclusive practices involve engaging individuals in typically occurring opportunities regardless of their ability. In an inclusive preschool, children with special needs participate in activities and opportunities with typically developing children. Adequate supports and adaptations should be provided for the children with special needs to promote full participation (Beattie, Jordan, & Algozzine, 2006).

An inclusive preschool practice may be challenging to implement considering the service structure, practice setting, role identities, and population-based approaches involved. Many processes and skills are involved in transforming practice from a segregated special classroom model to an integrated inclusive model incorporating gardening, dance, and community experiences. This chapter highlights the theoretical foundation for inclusive program development, the creation of rich therapeutic learning contexts for the children, and the skills needed to transition from a segregated practice to an integrated inclusive practice.

Theoretical Foundation

This project was grounded in human ecology principles. *Human ecology* refers to how people interact in and engage their social and physical environments and how those environments influence a person's development (Bronfenbrenner, 1979, 1999). The ecology of human performance model was our theoretical foundation for thinking about an inclusive practice (Dunn, Brown, & Youngstrom, 2003). It provided a framework for examining the reciprocal interactions of a person and their tasks with an emphasis on the "essential role of context on task performance" (p. 223). The ecology of human performance model explicitly states "occupational therapy practice involves promoting self-determination and inclusion of persons with disabilities in all aspects of society" (p. 236). The theoretical assumptions of self-determination and inclusion are not as explicitly stated in other occupational therapy theories as they are in the ecology of human performance. Another theoretical model that influenced our decision making was the ecology of human development (Bronfenbrenner, 1999).

These models emphasize dynamic reciprocal interaction between a person and the environment. Concepts that pervade these theories assume that (1) a person's participation in society is influenced by the person's perception of society; (2) if a person's perception is narrow, then the person's repertoire of responses and actions will also be narrow, whereas if the person's perception is broader, then the person's repertoire of responses and actions will be broader; and (3) a person has access to various environments and opportunities to participate in society (Bronfenbrenner, 1999; Dunn et al., 2003). Using these ecological concepts, we hypothesized that expanding the environmental opportunities at the preschool would broaden the children's repertoire of responses and perception of the world. Therefore, the goal of transitioning from a segregated practice to an inclusive occupational therapy practice was to increase the children's repertoire of behavioral responses by increasing their opportunities to learn.

The unique nature and variability of children's experiences led Bronfenbrenner (1999) to posit that learning activities should naturally become more complex over time; occur regularly over an extended period; and invite attention, exploration, manipulation, elaboration, and imagination. Dunn and colleagues also suggest strategies aimed at addressing a person's needs or modifying the context, including establishing, adapting, altering, preventing, and creating skills and new contexts for a person–environment match to promote optimal performance. These strategies can be aimed at either the internal processes of the child or the external processes surrounding the child (Dunn et al., 2003). Because the transition to an inclusive preschool practice included children with and without special needs and involved population-based services such as parent education and group-based interventions instead of individual interventions, the ecological concepts provided a grounding framework to create and adapt learning activities, routines, and environments.

Reviewing the Literature

Identifying and understanding a theoretical model was the first step in transitioning to an inclusive, population-oriented practice. A population-oriented practice is a practice directed at large groups of people (AOTA, 2008). In this case, the population was the entire preschool community and their families, which included children with special needs as well as typically developing children. Therefore, an inclusive philosophy of practice involved not merely considering the children with special needs but all the children in the preschool. The next step was to review the literature on inclusive practice. Literature in early childhood education, psychology, sociology, and occupational therapy was reviewed to examine the question, What is the evidence for optimizing outcomes within inclusive practices?

The literature challenged previously held concepts among practitioners about inclusion and learning. For example, we found that preschool children with mild–moderate disability showed gains in social and cognitive skills when in an inclusive environment (Buysse & Bailey, 1993; Garfinkle & Schwartz, 2002; Lee, Odom, & Loftin, 2007; Skinner, Buysse, & Bailey, 2004) but no difference in motor skill improvements whether in inclusive or segregated settings (Buysse & Bailey, 1993). The evidence on inclusive services for children with severe disabilities was much more mixed and inconclusive (Buysse & Bailey, 1993; Odom, 2000). Additionally, the literature suggested that children use different motor planning strategies for the same task when the task is presented in different contexts. Therefore, in essence, the task itself may be perceived by children as a different task in a different context (Ceci & Hembrooke, 1995).

The majority of literature on inclusion was found in the fields of education and psychology. A literature search in the *American Journal of Occupational Therapy* using the keyword *inclusion* resulted in six articles dating from 1995 to 2004. Five articles were documents or statements from AOTA (AOTA, 1995, 1996a, 1996b, 1999, 2004), and one article described a case study within a fully inclusive environment (Kellegrew & Allen, 1996). A review of the literature helped reduce any tentative feelings we had about inclusive and population-oriented approaches. Inclusive environments provide varied and reciprocal learning opportunities along with social integration to promote meaningful exploration of the physical and social environment for children with and without disabilities (Guralnick, 1999). Studies also reveal that natural learning environments and everyday experiences promote competence in both the social and nonsocial activities of children with special needs (Dunst, Hamby, Trivette, Raab, & Bruder, 2000; Dunst et al., 2001; Odom et al., 2004; Tsao et al., 2008). Therefore, children with special needs participating in inclusive and natural learning environments and experiences will be better prepared for social participation in the future.

The theoretical grounding and literature review helped us prepare a vision and direction for transforming practice from a segregated, adult-to-child, one-on-one therapy practice to an integrated, inclusive, adult-to-child and child-to-child, individual and social group therapy practice.

Creating a Context for Inclusive Programming

The following examples demonstrate how occupational therapy programming was responsible for creating and adapting the contexts of activities to establish opportunities for growth and learning (Dunn et al., 2003).

The examples include how a garden offered easily adapted experiences to meet diverse learning needs, how dance provided opportunities for children to establish new skills, and how community-based experiences were adapted to support a child's performance at museums.

Garden as Context

A garden was created as a learning space at the KenCrest preschool. The preschool is in a densely populated urban setting with a diverse racial population, including children who are from Hispanic, White, African-American, and Asian-American backgrounds. The preschool had green space around it, but the space was not used as a learning space due to unsafe paraphernalia, animal waste, and litter. The preschool community and occupational therapy students created a garden in this space to provide new learning opportunities for the children (see Figures 14.1 and 14.2). The occupational therapy students collaborated with the teachers to design and implement garden-related activities.

Ecological principles were incorporated in the garden activity experiences (Bronfenbrenner, 1999). The garden provided a context for variable and novel activities and experiences intended to invite attention, exploration, manipulation, elaboration, and imagination. The garden naturally became more complex over time as the vegetables and flowers grew and bloomed and birds and insects appeared in the space. Therapy-designed experiences such as nature scavenger hunts, bird-watching, vegetable picking, nature painting, and worm hunts were scheduled regularly. In addition, routine activities such as picnics, story time, watering days, and weeding days offered constant exposure to the garden (although we had to make sure the children were pulling weeds instead of vegetables or flowers). An example of the garden providing varied and novel activities included the natural growth of plants. In the fall, the children planted flower bulbs and prepared the garden beds for winter. In the winter, the children planted vegetable seeds and tracked plant growth, and in the summer they picked vegetables and flowers. The garden naturally changes and offers novel opportunities for children to explore their environment.

Dynamic activities and opportunities for children can facilitate unexpectedly complex performance. Ideishi, Idershi, Gandhi, and Yuen (2006) described a case when a preschool child with limited participation began to initiate social interactions during a nature scavenger hunt with his typically developing peers. The child would tug on his

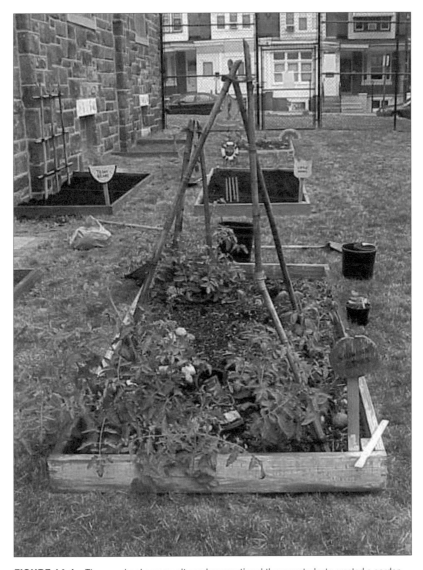

FIGURE 14.1. The preschool community and occupational therapy students created a garden in a previously unused green space.

search partner and make verbalizations to his partner and the teachers to request additional cue cards to find more objects in the garden. While searching, the child's cue card had a photograph of a wooden arbor lattice. In the child's search, he pointed at the metal window grill that had the same diagonal diamond shapes as the wooden arbor

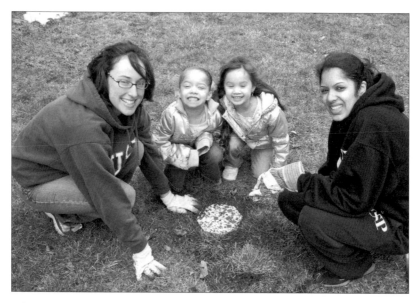

FIGURE 14.2. Occupational therapy students to create novel garden-related activities for the children.

lattice on the picture cue card. The child appeared to demonstrate his understanding of the spatial orientation of objects and shapes. Therapists and teachers had not noticed this child perform in other activities with this level of discrimination or attention to the environment.

The garden activity met the needs of diverse children. The typically developed children demonstrated searching skills and modeled environmental scanning, whereas the children with special needs participated at a level appropriate for their development. For example, a child with special needs may be just as engaged in searching and scanning or can follow a typically developed partner and participate in the excitement of matching picture cue cards with the garden item. The engagement of the child with special needs depends on the child, but the context and activity offer variability yet full participation in the experience. This case description doesn't imply that gardens facilitate performance skills. Nevertheless, this case suggests that when children are regularly exposed to contexts that have natural complexity rather than therapeutically contrived complexity, it promotes attention, exploration, manipulation, elaboration, and imagination (Bronfenbrenner, 1999). Therefore, occupational therapists can help create novel and rich contexts for therapeutic learning and engagement to enhance performance (Dunn et al., 2003).

Dance as Context

A dance program using the same learning principles as the garden program was created. Dance, as an art form, naturally becomes more complex over time as new steps are incorporated with older steps and dancers dance with or in front of others, wear a costume, or act out a scene through movement. Dance and movement activities were scheduled weekly through therapy-designed experiences such as ballet, imitating animal movements, animal yoga, and cultural dance (see Figure 14.3).

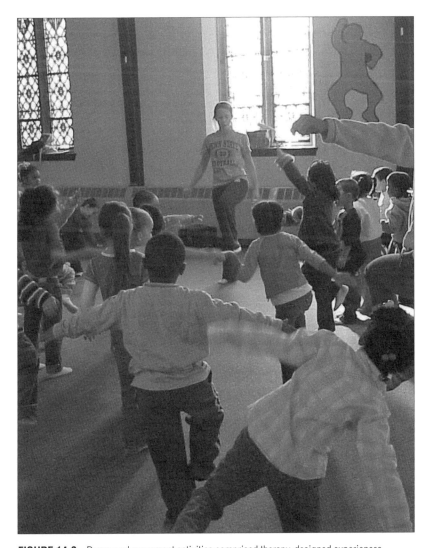

FIGURE 14.3. Dance and movement activities comprised therapy-designed experiences.

The dance program provided a context for social and personal expression. Lorenzo-Lasa, Ideishi, and Ideishi (2007) describe how children responded to movement variations and emotions when dancing like a hopping chicken versus dancing like a graceful swan or a regal horse. Children demonstrated the ability to modify and regulate their emotions according to the associated animal movement. They laughed and made jerky movements such as hopping like a funny chicken, yet they easily transitioned to the quiet and smooth movements of a graceful swan or to stiffer movements with their back and head pointing upward to display the confidence and the regal nature of a horse. The social and emotional associations of dance offer children opportunities to explore their movement expressions, elaborate on other emotions, and imagine dancing in different characters.

The dance activity met the needs of diverse children. The typically developed children demonstrated emotional character skills that the children with special needs were able to imitate or expand on. Children who weren't able to perform the characters of scenarios could clap to the music; match the excitement of movement with scarves, ribbons, and other dance artifacts; or play on drums. Again, the occupational therapists created novel and rich contexts for therapeutic learning and engagement to enhance performance (Dunn et al., 2003).

Museums and Aquariums as Context

Ecological principles encouraged us to expand our concept of *environment* from the immediate area to one that extends into and beyond the community. Developing a broader perception of the world to facilitate a broader repertoire of responses assumes the person has access to various environments and opportunities to participate in society (Bronfenbrenner, 1999; Dunn et al., 2003). From this concept emerged a museum and aquarium project. The project involved preparing the children for a community experience, encouraging parents and caregivers to participate in the preparatory activities and the subsequent community outings, taking the children to various community venues, and adapting or modifying the experience to promote optimal participation.

Museum and aquarium experiences become more complex as the children were able to more attend to the environments and explore them more deeply. Although museums and aquarium visits occur only a few times a year, related activities in collaboration with the museum and aquarium are planned regularly through therapy-designed experiences, such as an artist study of Vincent Van Gogh's and Georgia O'Keefe's flower paintings. Picture postcards and books with Van Gogh's and O'Keefe's paintings were displayed in the classroom, and children planted sunflowers in the garden, painting the actual flowers when they were in bloom in the garden. Other expressive arts and literacy experiences were planned throughout the year, culminating in a field trip to the art museum. The occupational therapists designed and adapted the activities for all children to participate at an appropriate level. Because there is a certain level of abstraction in Van Gogh's and O'Keefe's paintings, a variety of interpretations of each artist's flower paintings can be made. Additionally, all paintings, whether simple or complex or from typically developing children or children with special needs, can be deemed works of art. The regular exposure to Van Gogh and O'Keefe's paintings and art experiences prepared the children for their visit to the art museum and what they should look for at the museum. Because the children had developed scavenger hunt skills throughout the year in garden activities, a scavenger hunt activity based on the museum paintings took place. The familiar activity provided self-direction and goals for the children's engagement.

Other examples of integrating school activities with community experiences included the museum and aquarium bringing their community outreach program to the preschool. The outreach programs introduced the children to objects, animals, and activities that they might see or experience on future visits to the museum and aquarium. The outreach programs can introduce the children to new experiences and objects in a safe and familiar environment (i.e., at school). Additional preparation included the teachers, therapists, and parents reading social stories about the museum and aquarium that described situations the children might encounter at these venues. A *social story* "describes a situation, skill, or concept in terms of relevant social cues, perspectives, and common responses" (Gray, 2004, p. 2). These social stories familiarize a child with certain situations to promote participation or facilitate transitioning to new experiences. The museum and aquarium staff and a health team that included occupational therapists, a pediatrician, a speech pathologist, and a psychologist made special sensory maps of the museum and aquarium to match each child's sensory preferences (Ross, Ideishi, Jackel, & Jones, 2009; Thach & Ideishi, 2009).

The novelty of museum and aquarium objects and animals invites attention, exploration, manipulation, and imagination. These dynamic activities and opportunities for children can facilitate unexpected performance. Thach and Ideishi (2009) found children with autism actually touched aquarium animals, to the surprise of the children's parents, teachers, and therapists. This preconception of the adults about the children may indicate that adults can inadvertently limit children's participation, engagement, and exploration. The aquarium example highlights the dynamic and unexpected outcomes that can occur when children with special needs are supported, given choices to engage in novel experiences, and provided opportunities to explore and participate in natural environments.

Skills Occupational Therapists Need to Create an Inclusive Context

The process of transforming a therapeutic practice from a segregated, adult-to-child and one-on-one interaction–based therapy to an integrated, inclusive one with more child-to-child interactions than adult-to-child–facilitated ones required a different set of skills than the therapist's previously used. The garden, dance, and museum examples involved changing the occupational therapists' role to include creating and expanding environmental opportunities, expanding their consultative services, and broadening the therapists' concept of resources to include grants, business connections to obtain donations and services, and partnerships with academic, cultural, and community organizations.

The occupational therapists' role change involved understanding that inclusive therapeutic impact often occurs without the presence of the therapist. This should not be interpreted as the occupational therapist not doing anything. The occupational therapist created and adapted the therapeutic context and activities. In doing this, the occupational therapist designed environments for learning that occur over time instead of during discrete therapeutic sessions. The adaptations that are incorporated into the environment are naturally occurring adaptations such as growing plants, designing or making easily donned and changeable costumes for dancing, or gathering picture postcards to display in the classroom for self-initiated exploration of visual images.

These contextual adaptations support the child not only during discrete therapeutic sessions but also during the teacher's lesson activities and the child's self-initiated exploration. The therapist needs to constantly try to predict the children's changing interests and meaning and plan accordingly. By designing an environment that encourages joint and reciprocal engagement, the occupational therapist is attending not only to the child with special needs who is on the caseload but also to the entire class, the other children, the teacher, and the parents.

Wesley, Buysse, and Skinner (2001) found that practitioners in early intervention and early childhood education often understood that consultative services were similar to providing direct intervention, and consultants were expected to fix problems rather than engage in a collaborative process to address perceived barriers. Consultation is indirect and involves joint problem solving to achieve a particular outcome.

We embraced the idea that designing and creating environments for therapeutic impact and engagement (when done specifically to create adaptations for a child with special needs) *is* a consultative process. Often the individual therapeutic outcome for a child is to provide opportunities for the child to engage in activities promoting child-to-child interactions and self-directed exploration and engagement. The child's self-discovery becomes the outcome rather than an adult determining what the child's actions should be. Designing these types of opportunities requires effective communication among the stakeholders, such as therapist, child, and parent, to understand the child and the family's values and interests. It also requires communicating and interacting with the teacher to ensure that the environment is consistent with lesson planning and educational curriculum. In addition, occupational therapists' participation in the teacher's lesson planning ensures that the environment meets the needs of all the children, whether typically developing or not. Occupational therapy consultation in inclusive settings ensures optimal participation of the child with special needs but also requires the occupational therapist to perceive, understand, and participate in the development of the entire classroom environment.

Another important skill for the occupational therapist is writing grants. These unique therapeutic programs are not necessarily within the general operating budget of a preschool program. These programs, as well as other inclusive programs such as photography activities and parent education, were paid for with external funds. From an ecological perspective, the broader economic and political environment of funding for early childhood education and therapy services may not necessarily fully support unique, creative, and innovative programming. Therefore, seeking external funds to implement these ideas was an important professional development initiative. To date, we have obtained approximately $25,000 of external funding to support these programs.

Implementing these inclusive therapeutic programs required partnering with diverse individuals and groups. Parent participation connected the preschool, community, and home experiences, reinforcing ideas and experiences. University service-learning programs were key to providing additional human resources to support activity programs so that programming wasn't only implemented during therapy sessions. Occupational therapy, health science, and art education students support these programs 12 months a year. Individuals from the local arts community, including dancers and musicians, are supported through the external funds to help develop arts curricula and implement short-term artist residencies. These artist residencies are 3 to 6 weeks long. The artists work directly with the children to engage in a performance art once or twice per week during the residency. The therapists and service-learning students create the appropriate adaptations for the children with special needs to participate in the experience. The community-outreach programs of local institutions, such as theater and dance companies, museums, and aquariums, come to the preschool two to three times per year as part of the children's introduction to community experiences. In addition, these outreach programs offer opportunities for the children to attend live performances at the ballet, theater, and orchestra. Identifying, connecting, building, and sustaining community partnerships and resources are a hallmark of the inclusive therapeutic programming and should be actively sought out.

Conclusion

Within the structure of research, the purpose and intent of Living Life To Its Fullest™ is present as both researchers and clients work toward a more occupation-rich life. An occupational therapy practitioner may have to examine and develop new roles, new service structures, and new therapy partners. The world is rich with opportunities and experiences that stimulate a child's mind and body.

Inclusive therapeutic programming is a rich and dynamic experience that is often unpredictable, but as a result of the unpredictability, children with special needs often present unexpected adaptive responses that are "typical" responses within the natural flow of the experience and environment. At this inclusive preschool, the therapeutic programming includes the children's peers, the outdoors, and the community—not merely as a context for therapy but also as actors and agents to facilitate therapeutic change.

References

American Occupational Therapy Association. (1995). Statement—Nondiscrimination and inclusion regarding members of the occupational therapy professional community. *American Journal of Occupational Therapy, 49*, 1009.

American Occupational Therapy Association. (1996a). Occupational therapy: A profession in support of full inclusion. *American Journal of Occupational Therapy, 50*, 855.

American Occupational Therapy Association. (1996b). White Paper—The role of the occupational therapy practitioner in the implementation of full inclusion. *American Journal of Occupational Therapy, 50*, 856–857.

American Occupational Therapy Association. (1999). Occupational therapy's commitment to nondiscrimination and inclusion [Position Paper]. *American Journal of Occupational Therapy, 53*, 598.

American Occupational Therapy Association. (2004). Occupational therapy's commitment to nondiscrimination and inclusion. *American Journal of Occupational Therapy, 58,* 668.

American Occupational Therapy Association. (2008). Occupational therapy practice framework: Domain and process (2nd ed.). *American Journal of Occupational Therapy, 62*, 625–683.

Beattie, J., Jordan, L., & Algozzine, B. (2006). *Making inclusion work: Effective practices for all teachers.* Thousand Oaks, CA: Corwin Press/Sage Publications.

Bronfenbrenner, U. (1979). *The ecology of human development.* Cambridge, MA: Harvard University Press.

Bronfenbrenner, U. (1999). Environments in developmental perspective: Theoretical and operational models. In S. L. Friedman & T. D. Wachs (Eds.), *Measuring environment across the life span: Emerging methods and concepts* (pp. 3–25). Washington, DC: American Psychological Association.

Buysse, V., & Bailey, D. B. (1993). Behavioral and developmental outcomes in young children with disabilities in integrated and segregated settings: A review of comparative studies. *Journal of Special Education, 26*, 434–461.

Ceci, S. J., & Hembrooke, H. A. (1995). A bioecological model of intellectual development. In P. Moen, G. H. Elder, & K. Lüsher (Eds.), *Examining lives in context: Perspectives on the ecology of human development* (pp. 312–328). Washington, DC: American Psychological Association.

Dunn, W., Brown, C., & Youngstrom, M. J. (2003). Ecological model of occupation. In P. Kramer, J. Hinojosa, & C. B. Royeen (Eds.), *Perspectives on human occupation: Participation in life* (pp. 222–263). Philadelphia: Lippincott, Williams & Wilkins.

Dunst, C. J., Bruder, M. B., Trivette, C. M., Hamby, D., Raab, D., & McLean, M. (2001). Characteristics and consequences of everyday natural learning opportunities. *Topics in Early Childhood Special Education, 21*, 68–92.

Dunst, C. J., Hamby, D., Trivette, C. M., Raab, M., & Bruder, M. B. (2000). Everyday family and community life and children's naturally occurring learning opportunities. *Journal of Early Intervention, 23*, 151–164.

Garfinkle, A. N., & Schwartz, I. S. (2002). Peer imitation: Increasing social interactions of children with autism and other developmental disabilities in inclusive preschool classrooms. *Topics in Early Childhood Special Education,* *22,* 26–38.

Gray, C. (2004). Social Stories, 10.0. *Jenison Autism Journal, 15,* 1–28. Obtain additional information on Social Stories from http://www.thegraycenter.org/

Guralnick, M. (1999). The nature and meaning of social integration for young children with mild developmental delays in inclusive settings. *Journal of Early Intervention, 22,* 70–86.

Ideishi, S. K., Ideishi, R. I., Gandhi, T., & Yuen, L. (2006). Inclusive preschool outdoor play environments. *School System Special Interest Section Quarterly,* *13*(2), 1–4.

Kellegrew, D. H., & Allen, D. (1996). Occupational therapy in full-inclusion classrooms: A case study from the Moorpark model. *American Journal of Occupational Therapy, 50,* 718–724.

KenCrest. (2009). *Services for children.* Retrieved January 28, 2010, from http://www.kencrest.org/services_for_children.htm

Kramer, P., Ideishi, R. I., Kearney, P. K., Cohen, M. E., Ames, J. O., Shea, G. B., et al. (2007). Achieving curricular themes through learner-centered teaching. *Occupational Therapy in Health Care, 21,* 185–198.

Lee, S., Odom, S. L., & Loftin, R. (2007). Social engagement with peers and stereotypic behavior of children with autism. *Journal of Positive Behavior Interventions, 9*(2), 67–79.

Lorenzo-Lasa, R., Ideishi, R. I., & Ideishi, S. K. (2007). Facilitating preschool learning and movement through dance. *Early Childhood Education Journal,* *35,* 25–31.

Odom, S. L. (2000). Preschool inclusion: What we know and where we go from here. *Topics in Early Childhood Special Education, 20,* 20–27.

Odom, S. L.,Vitztum, J., Wolery, R., Lieber, J., Sandall, S., Hanson, M. J., et al. (2004). Preschool inclusion in the United States: A review of research from an ecological systems perspective. *Journal of Research in Special Educational Needs, 4,* 17–49.

Ross, W., Ideishi, R., Jackel, R., & Jones, A. (2009, August). *Museums and autism spectrum disorder.* Paper presented at the National Autism Conference, State College, PA.

Skinner, M. L, Buysse, V., & Bailey, D. B. (2004). Effects of age and developmental status of partners on play of preschoolers with disabilities. *Journal of Early Intervention, 26*(3), 194–203.

Thach, K., & Ideishi, R. I. (2009, April). *Access and social participation at the aquarium for children with autism spectrum disorder.* Poster presented at the meeting of the American Occupational Therapy Association, Houston, TX.

Tsao, L., Odom, S. L., Buysse, V., Skinner, M., West, T., & Vitztum-Komanecki, J. (2008). Social participation of children with disabilities in inclusive preschool programs: Program typology and ecological features. *Exceptionality,* *16*(3), 125–140.

Wesley, P. W., Buysse, V., & Skinner, D. (2001). Early interventionists' perspectives on professional comfort as consultants. *Journal of Early Intervention, 24*(2), 112–128.

CHAPTER 15

Journey to Home

Ami Dholakia, *OTR/L*

Potomac Center is a 230-bed skilled nursing facility located in Arlington, Virginia, that provides both inpatient and outpatient rehab services. There is never a dull day here as the therapists treat various complex medical conditions and comorbidities. Although the therapists treat quite complex conditions, they never forget the core principles of patient-focused, client-centered treatment. We do not just treat the medical condition; we treat the whole person, trying to understand the occupations, roles, and interests that define who our clients are.

One unique individual comes to mind when I think of remarkable outcomes. The thought of her still gives us a sense of pride and hope and the knowledge that we can achieve the best functional outcomes for our residents. No matter what hurdles lie ahead of us and our clients, we can achieve living life to its fullest.

Ms. Martez was a young woman who came to the Potomac Center in July 2008. She had a 3-month hospitalization due to meningioma, which led to a craniotomy. She had been confined to bed since the procedure. She was incontinent of both bowel and bladder and could not speak. Even the simplest tasks, such as washing her face with a washcloth or turning from side to side in bed, required extensive assistance. The light at the end of the tunnel seemed far away.

Prior to her prolonged hospitalization, Ms. Martez had quite an active life. She was a housewife with two young sons, one 10 years old and another 9 months old. She enjoyed socializing and was active in the community. She missed her family dearly while she was in the hospital. She longed to be able to hold her baby and to cook the delicious El Salvadorian cuisine that her family enjoyed so much.

There is a saying that it isn't the result that matters most, it's the means we use to get there. In the beginning of this journey the therapists involved had to settle for baby steps in Ms. Martez's treatment. Treatment sessions were conducted at bedside, one-on-one. Sitting at the edge of the bed with two people assisting her was an achievement, as were tasks like speaking one or two words. Ms. Martez's treatment required great teamwork, as many of her sessions were cotreated.

Over time, we noted that she had improved activity tolerance, strength, and range of motion. She could once again perform tasks such as feeding herself, speaking more sentences with clear quality, putting her shirt on, and standing with a walker, and walking a few steps. Modalities such as electrical stimulation were used to alleviate pain in her neck and upper back as well as improve strength. She was also fitted with ankle orthotics. A few weeks later, she was able to walk further, independently propel herself in the wheelchair, and bathe and dress herself with little assistance. She developed better upper- and lower-body strength and had fewer complaints of pain. Because she was quite a sociable individual, she enjoyed therapy groups. She had a great rapport with the rehabilitation staff as well as the residents. She motivated and encouraged other residents. When she wasn't occupied with her therapy sessions, she regularly attended various activities held by the recreational therapy department. She became an ardent fan of bingo.

Although she was progressing in therapy quite well, she still felt incomplete. She felt as though her children were growing up without her. Her husband had been juggling a full-time job in construction as well as taking care of their two young sons. She longed to resume the roles of housewife and mother. More than anything, she just wanted to be *home*.

Treatment focused on getting Ms. Martez to return home and resume these roles. Physical therapy became more aggressive with balance retraining, car transfers, stair climbing, and transitioning to the use of a cane and walker. Occupational therapy began to incorporate homemaking tasks such as cooking, light household tasks, and even child care. A doll was given to her and strapped with an 8-pound cuff weight. Her assignment was to care for this doll and carry it with her everywhere she went to simulate taking care of her baby, who weighed around 20 pounds at the time. She took good care of this new "baby," stroking its hair and singing to it. Every day we therapists witnessed fragments of her self—a self that had been shattered by her long illness—slowly come back together.

Finally, after she had been with us for 3 months, we felt that it was safe for her to return home. Her father came from El Salvador to stay with her for 6 months to make the transition easier. Her son had become a young man during this time, and he assumed responsibility for many of the household chores. All of the medical equipment she needed had been ordered and would be delivered to her home soon. This journey we experienced with her lasted about 3 months.

Saying good-bye wasn't easy. It felt as though we were watching a young adult leave home for the first time. We all were so incredibly proud of her, but we didn't want her to leave.

CHAPTER 16

OT Smells Like Cookies and Sounds Like Laughter

Melissa Winkle, *OTR/L*

Prior to occupational therapy school, I volunteered at a veteran's hospital in the physical therapy department and enjoyed my position. I recall the routine of walking down the long corridor observing dismayed patients and fast moving staff. People were crowded in alcoves waiting for appointments, for visitors, and perhaps for the time to pass. One day seemed significantly different than the rest. I remember seeing a woman with lymphedema, unable to support her own body weight, crying because she just wanted to take a shower. There were people hovering over emesis basins, sick from vertigo, medications, and procedures; others with enormous bedsores being transferred into the hydrotherapy tanks; and grown men becoming angry or giving up in response to routine physical therapy activities such as weight bearing and strength training. One man sat in his wheelchair with tears in his eyes quietly reaching for a blanket to cover the fact that he had soiled himself. His family members appeared defeated, as they probably wondered if this was ultimately what the future held. The process of rehab was difficult, and while people were in pain and wanted to give up, I knew it would be worthwhile in the end, and I hoped they knew it, too.

I returned from lunch thinking that the halls seemed more crowded and the patients seemed more dismayed than usual. I wondered if the feeling in my gut was normal and hoped that it was transient. Something was in the air, and I felt as if I was on the outside looking in. In an instant, I found myself ducking into an unfamiliar doorway to get out of the way of a gurney that whizzed by with a man screaming because he had "led troops in the war, and nobody would let him go to his own @#$%! home to live on his own." I wondered what happened that this man could fight for our country, for my freedom, and now, could not win the battle to live independently in his own home. I stood against the wall, away from the sea of open wounds and body fluids, and was taken aback by the energy of it all. I closed my eyes and thought "breathe," and so I did.

However, the sounds and smells through the unfamiliar door would forever change my career path. I noticed a patient whose belly bounced when he laughed. He stood, carefully using the brakes of his walker so he could bend just enough to see in the oven window. "Mr. Johnson, do you need to sit and take a break?" asked the OT. "And risk burning my cookies? No thanks!" he said. This was the same man who, just hours before, refused to stand or do exercises in the PT gym. And he now refused to sit because his cookies might burn? He turned to another patient who had a pile of coins and a calculator in front of him and stated, "Smells good, huh?" He paused, exchanged whispers with the occupational therapist, and then continued, "46 cents for you, airman." It took three tries before the airman could accurately count, but he finally purchased the cookie. The men sat with each other and the occupational therapy staff and laughed over cookies. They were in rehab, they had cookies, and they were happy.

Cookies? That is what motivated one man with a physical disability to stand longer than he ever had before and another man with a traumatic brain injury to count money three times? Clearly, the cookies possessed a higher power.

The following week I started my rotation in the occupational therapy department. When one of the physical therapists asked why I was making the change, I thought about the smell of cookies and the sound of laughter. "You know you will have to do bathroom training, right?" he asked. I was not sure what that meant, but explained that I was armed with whoopee cushions and toilet paper. I could hold my own.

It was a transition time at the end of my first week in the occupational therapy department. Individuals were exiting sessions as others entered. The therapists were detailing home plans with caregivers for individuals going home for the weekend. In the midst of the chaos, an older gentleman looked me in the eye and called out, "Honey, I have to go to the bathroom." He was using his feet and hands to move the wheelchair into the bathroom, but he did not yet have the strength to transfer. I called back to him, "I'll go find someone. Hang in there, I'll be right back." But everyone was busy. He began to sob and called out "Please, I can't wait, I need help. Please, I don't want to soil myself." That is when I recognized him as the man from the previous week who had soiled himself in the hallway. Predicting the outcome, he began crying and pleading for my help. I had seen transfers done a million times and had assisted with a handful of two-person transfers. Could I do this? Family members did it, women half the size of their loved ones did it. "Please!" he cried. In one blur of movement, we managed clothing and transferred. And it was just in time. He continued crying and would not let me go. I was frozen, not knowing the right response to this awkward situation. Finally, he found words and said "I'm not in charge of my own dignity right now. I used to be someone important, and now I can't make it to the bathroom. Thank you for helping me keep my dignity." He had felt as if he had nothing left. No dignity, no self-worth, and little strength to get it back. I wondered if this is what the PT meant? If bathroom transfer training was all it took to give someone a sense of self-worth, sign me up!

Five years later, I completed occupational therapy school and was working with a young man who had a traumatic brain injury. During the evaluation, he was not able to communicate verbally, but it was clear he understood. His family described him before the injury as a fast-moving, quick-thinking, practical joker. He loved life and lived to get responses out of people. It had been just over a year since the injury, and he had been receiving physical therapy and occupational therapy, but was becoming difficult to engage in therapeutic activities. The family agreed that transfers and balance were the two greatest goals. Could this rookie occupational therapist make it happen?

Three months later, it was time to train the family with some home strategies. My client slowly handed them a brown bag that contained the mystery equipment necessary for the home exercise plan. The family was pleasantly surprised when we demonstrated how to use the whoopee cushion during transitional movements. He had to take breaks for incessant laughter, but his strength was coming back. His standing balance plan included a gait belt and rolls of toilet paper with explicit instructions on how to toilet paper his brother's car. He and his family were once again laughing and engaged in a plan.

Sometimes people need to find their dignity and their sense of self, even if it is on a toilet. Sometimes they and their families need permission to laugh, even in the presence of disability. Occupational therapy is individual-specific and has few boundaries. We provide people with the tools to help themselves become independent. When people ask me why I finally chose occupational therapy, I explain that OT smells like cookies and sounds like laughter.

CHAPTER **17**

Living Independently With Rheumatoid Arthritis

Rebecca D. Nesbitt, *MS, OTR/L*

Mrs. Irene Paine is a remarkable woman whom I have known since August 2006. She is a resident of Aldersgate Retirement Community in Charlotte, North Carolina, and has severe rheumatoid arthritis with multiple joint replacements, a history of numerous fractures, and severe osteoarthritis and osteoporosis. She has very limited use of her hands, has decreased balance, and uses a rolling walker for mobility within her apartment and a power wheelchair outside her apartment. Most people with Mrs. Paine's health conditions would require an assisted-living or skilled level of care, but through a lot of hard work and frequent therapy intervention, Mrs. Paine is still able to live independently in her home.

Mrs. Paine's story shows the positive effect occupational therapy can have in a continuing care retirement community setting where therapists can treat residents for outpatient therapy in a traditional "gym" setting, within their community and within their home. In the 3 years since Mrs. Paine moved to Aldersgate, she has had frequent outpatient therapy intervention, as well as physical therapy and speech therapy.

Mrs. Paine's occupational therapy resulted in home modifications that allowed her to maintain independence in her apartment. Interventions within Mrs. Paine's apartment included customized knobs on her washer and dryer made with splinting material, customized switches in her kitchen so she can easily turn appliances on and off, an extension on her keys so she can turn them in the lock, touch switches on her lamps so they can easily be turned on and off, window handles installed so that she can easily open and close her windows, and lowering her closet racks so that she can reach to hang her clothing. She has additional adaptations to increase accessibility to her bathroom, including grab bars, a nonslip pad on the floor of shower, a shower seat, a bedside commode, and a bidet. Occupational therapists also assisted Mrs. Paine with developing a safe method to access the swimming pool and a pool exercise program. Mrs. Paine participates in a facility-sponsored supervised swim program twice per week and reports a resulting decrease in arthritic pain.

Most recently, Mrs. Paine developed increased hand and wrist contractures, further limiting her fine motor coordination. Crystal Sottile, the new staff occupational therapist in the building, had an idea for contracture management and fitted dynamic splints for both of Mrs. Paine's wrists and hands. Together, Crystal and Mrs. Paine developed a wearing schedule, and Mrs. Paine is able to don and doff the splints at an independent level—no small feat for someone with severe hand deformities.

During her time at Aldersgate, Mrs. Paine has battled through many illnesses, fractures, and increased complications from her rheumatoid arthritis. Mrs. Paine's story shows the positive effect occupational therapy has in a continuing care retirement community setting like Aldersgate, where residents are encouraged to maintain their independence and therapy practitioners are able to work in a resident's home to continually adapt items as the resident ages in place. The resident and therapists develop a close relationship, and this in-depth knowledge of a resident's strengths and limitations enables the therapeutic process to result in interventions that increase participation and quality of life for the resident. The combination of therapeutic intervention and Mrs. Paine's desire to remain independent has created this remarkable outcome. This is a true success story of independence.

CHAPTER 18

To Live Again

Charisma Quiambao-Fernandez, *OTR/L*
Patricia Mazur, *MPT*

> *"Reach for the fullness of human life. If you but touch it, it will fascinate. We live it all, but few live it knowingly."*
> —*Goethe,* Faust, *1881/2000*

Rosemarie lay in her bed, dependent for all activities of daily living due to exacerbation of congestive heart failure and pulmonary disease. After 10 months and a few tries at therapy, she had resigned herself to this life until her new roommate, Jean, moved in. Jean was very ill, very weak, and had difficulty breathing. She was dependent for all activities, too.

When Jean started therapy, she struggled. But her occupational therapist and physical therapist would not give up and neither would Jean. The three of them pushed on and soon Jean was transferring, walking, dressing, and becoming independently mobile. After seeing all that Jean had accomplished, Rosemarie knew that she wanted the chance to try therapy again. Rosemarie requested physical and occupational therapy evaluations.

At the evaluation, she told her physical therapist, Pat Mazur, and her occupational therapist, Charisma Fernandez, "I want to live my life again." Rosemarie had no idea how much those words would change her life. Rosemarie would need to battle fatigue, weakness, pain, and frustration. Her therapists used multiple approaches to get her through the ups and down of a taxing recovery.

On her first day of therapy she stood beside her bed with maximum assistance of two therapists and trunk flexion of 20 degrees for 30 seconds. Rosemarie had climbed her first mountain in 10 months. Rosemarie was frightened and fatigued but her therapists reminded her of the day she told them, "I want to live my life." With renewed motivation and strength, treatment continued. Two weeks later, Rosemarie walked five steps to the restroom; she cried. Two months later, the once frail, broken woman, who had lain in bed for 10 months, dressed herself, used the restroom, and walked down the halls of Coquina Center using her walker with her therapists by her side.

Rosemarie now focuses on the possibilities and fullness of her life. She is focused on her upcoming discharge and returning home to her husband, George. Rosemarie now embraces her potential and the fullness of human life—knowingly.

Reference

Goethe, J. W. (2000). *Faust: A tragedy.* New York, NY: W. W. Norton & Company. (original work published 1881)

CHAPTER **19**

"Just Call Me the Wii Man"

Patricia Larkin-Upton,
PT, MPT, MS, CWS

Michael, 52 years old, was admitted to Laurel Center Skilled
Nursing and Rehabilitation Facility (LC) on January 12, 2007, with
chronic anemia and acute renal failure. He had come to LC from another
skilled nursing facility in the area, where he had been receiving total
assistance and been confined to bed since June 2006. Michael's medical
history included hyperkalemia, Methicillin-resistant staphylococcus
aureus, sleep apnea with a need for a continuous positive airway
pressure, gastrointestinal bleeding, hypertension, peripheral vascular
disease, right-below-knee amputation, seizure disorders, deep vein
thrombosis in his right arm, gastric reflux, depression, obesity, anxiety,
diabetes mellitus, hyperlipidemia, cerebral atrophy, osteoarthritis, and
coccygodynia.

Upon evaluation by physical therapy and occupational therapy
at LC, Michael was found to be dependent for all movement and care.
He was very depressed and unmotivated due to his past struggles to get
rid of his pain, get out of bed and get home, all without success. He also
had multiple open wounds on his left foot and coccyx, multiple contractures of his arms and legs, poor strength, poor fine motor control,
and severe coccyx pain and was unable to sit up more than 30 minutes
in a reclined wheelchair without excruciating pain.

Michael was immediately treated by physical and occupational
therapy with modalities like short wave diathermy and electrical stimulation for his pain, contractures, and wounds; assessed for appropriate
seating and positioning; and began mobility, transfer, coordination, balance, dining, activities of daily living, and strength training. With the
help of his rehabilitation team, he made good progress and regained
the ability to move himself in bed, sit up alone, feed himself easily, and
sit in a wheelchair for more than 2 hours at a time. In addition, his
wounds healed completely.

During his stay at LC, Michael continued to develop new medical problems, sending him back to the acute care hospital several times.

After each hospital stay, Michael returned to his prehospital level of function with the help of his rehabilitation team. But, Michael was becoming more and more depressed and began to plateau with traditional therapy interventions.

That's when Michael's occupational therapist, Lori Lanza, OTR/L, introduced him to Wii boxing as an adjunct to his other treatments. It worked! Michael's mood brightened, his strength increased, his pain lessened, and his motivation increased. Michael was able to progress to an independent slide board transfer, independent wheelchair mobility, and even stand in the parallel bars with the help of his therapists.

Michael originally had only one goal, which was to lie in his skilled nursing facility bed without being in pain. But more than 2 years after his first hospital admittance with no return home—and with the never-say-die attitude of his rehabilitation team—Michael was finally able to return home to his wife and two young children with a renewed sense of life.

CHAPTER 20

Making Meaning to the End

Heather Javaherian, *OTD, OTR/L*

It was Valentine's Day. My husband, Hamid, had been hospitalized for nearly 2½ months with numerous life-threatening complications from surgery. Eight months earlier our world had been turned upside down when he was diagnosed with Stage IV gastric adenocarcinoma. What we initially thought was a bleeding ulcer was stomach cancer. It was in the advanced stages and required the doctors to remove two-thirds of Hamid's stomach. Our children—Ariyana, 20 months old, and Afshin, just 1 month old—were home with my parents who were a 1½ hours' drive away. They came to visit us nearly every other day. Each time I watched them drive away, my heart broke. I was desperate to be with my children, to be home again, to wake up from this terrible dream. But that was not my path; my husband, my soul mate, was dying.

Finding Meaning Through Occupation

I knew that I had a choice to make our last months meaningful, whether it was here in the hospital or at home on hospice. The mundane routine of the hospital, with procedures, medications, and boredom, deprives people of their everyday occupations. I have been an occupational therapist for 12 years and knew that participation in meaningful occupations brings hope and a sense of purpose to one's life. Occupation is the "primary means by which we organize the worlds in which we live…[and gives] shape to our daily lives" (Hasselkus, 2006, p. 627). Hamid and I needed to find meaning; we needed to engage in occupation together to help us reconnect and share our love and hope.

Through our 2½ months at the hospital, I saw Hamid's soul slipping away even faster than his body. It seemed that we had little to talk about except the next time Ariyana and Afshin would visit. I realized that it was only when we were *doing occupations* that we were able to break free of the cancer and the grip of the hospital environment. Finding meaning through occupation at the hospital was necessary for both of us to survive.

I remembered sitting by Hamid's bedside 2 months earlier as he lay in the intensive care unit fighting for his life. I felt so helpless as I watched his chest rise and fall with the ventilator. I needed to do something with my hands. When my mom and dad came down later that day they took me to the store where I bought yarn. I went back to the intensive care unit and took my seat beside Hamid. I started knitting and praying. Every so often I would pause and touch Hamid, talk to him, but then I would knit and pray with each row that he would live, he would see his son born, that we would make more memories before God took him home. Looking back, we lived Mary Reilly's (1962) words that "man, through the use of his hands as they are energized by mind and will, can influence the state of his own health" (p. 88) through my knitting, and the meaningful occupations we created on our journey toward his death.

Anticipating that this Valentine's Day would be our last one together, I wanted it to be special even though we were in an oncology unit in the hospital. I talked to the nurses and began making plans. Hamid and I took a walk around the unit, and the charge nurse set everything up so the room would be ready when we came back. As we walked into the room, there was a candle glowing on his bedside table, a small gift bag with a movie in it, a large TV and DVD player, and a delicate cloth rose. As we walked past the bed that I slept in, I hit play on my laptop, and our wedding song started. I remember it took a few moments for Hamid to realize the significance of the song and then when he looked up at me, I asked him to dance. We stood there, him in his hospital gown and IVs, dancing ever so gently and crying together as we celebrated what we knew was a love that would transcend all time.

Time to Go Home and Live

Hamid was home on hospice. We had many hard days, but with the hospice team's care and dedication to quality of life there were also many great days. One day while he was in the midst of a round of steroids and feeling good, I was talking to my sister and her husband who wanted to figure out how we could get Hamid to the beach. I thanked them but said it just wasn't possible with all of his IV medications and his physical state. He was able to walk with assistance but only for short distances and then he would need to rest. He usually went downstairs only once a day and that tired him. But now my mind started turning as I thought about how much we loved the beach and how the only time he had been outside of our home during the past 5 months had been to go to the hospital in San Diego. Occupational therapists think out of the box and adapt situations to meet people's needs and abilities. Why should going to the beach be off-limits?

I knew Hamid couldn't walk at the beach, but I knew he could ride there. So I rented a convertible for the weekend. On Saturday, I told Hamid he had to get dressed because we had a surprise. He kept wanting to know what it was, and then in a fearful voice told me that he could not leave the house. I was a little nervous that he might not want to go, but I just smiled and told him not to worry. With the help of my parents, we put his wheelchair, IV medications, dressing changes, and sun hat in the car. As I helped him with his sponge bath that morning, he kept asking what the surprise was—I laughed and told him that he sounded just like a little kid at Christmas. He was so excited. He put on pants and a shirt for the first time in over 5 months. He looked and felt like a new person who had a *purpose*—to see what the surprise was! We came downstairs and Ariyana exclaimed, "Baba, baba, come see the surprise."

He smiled, and we all walked outside. He was so surprised and initially said, "You bought a convertible?!" Laughing, I told him no, and walked with him to the car so that we could go for a ride. We waved to my parents and the kids as we drove away.

It was one of those perfect spring days with a bright blue sky. We drove through the mountains enjoying the beautiful scenery and fresh air. It gave us time to talk, to really talk about our love, our life together. Hamid always loved driving; though he couldn't drive himself, this was a way for him to experience it again and, even if only for a few hours, escape from the cancer. It was hard to really talk with Hamid during those last months. It was only during times like this, doing something meaningful, that the walls came down, and we were once again just two young people in love who together could face anything.

We drove to Newport Beach both wearing our big sun hats, and then down to Balboa Island where we remembered many dinners at the pub on the corner. We rode across the ferry in our car and even saw a seal swimming nearby. Afterward, we drove down the Pacific Coast Highway to Laguna Beach. We pulled off several times just to look at the ocean, listen to the waves, and watch people swim and walk in the sand. At Laguna Beach we headed home, driving again through the mountains with the sun shining down on us. I asked Hamid if he minded if I stopped for ice cream. He knew how much I loved ice cream, but I wanted to check with him as he hadn't been able to eat now for over 5 months. Holding my hand, he said of course, so I quickly ordered an ice cream. He snuck a lick of ice cream, but in bending down he got some on the tip of his sun hat. I started laughing. As I tried to point to the ice cream now dripping off his sun hat, we both laughed until we cried. Still laughing, I took a bite of the cone and then realized that I too had leaned too far forward and had ice cream dripping off my hat. It felt so good to laugh together.

All of this was only possible through occupation. We stopped being afraid of Hamid being sick and just reveled in the fact that he was alive and we were together. I know that being an occupational therapist helped me to make meaning in our last year together. Creating meaningful occupations gave us a time to share our love, to laugh, to be grateful for our blessings, and to have quality time with our children. It could have been very different. I even think Hamid would not have lived as long if he hadn't had those meaningful occupations to look forward to. Although he had cancer and was on hospice, Hamid was much more than that—*we* were much more than that. We were alive, and we were a family living each day, thankful for each moment.

References

Hasselkus, B. (2006). The world of everyday occupation: Real people, real lives [Eleanor Clarke Slagle Lecture]. *American Journal of Occupational Therapy, 60,* 627–640.

Reilly, M. (1962). Occupational therapy can be one of the great ideas of 20th-century medicine [Eleanor Clarke Slagle Lecture]. *American Journal of Occupational Therapy, 16,* 87–105.

Part IV

Insiders

CHAPTER **21**

Always the OT, Never the Patient

Brenna Meixner, *MOT, OTR/L*

Being a therapist and waking up as a patient is a frightening, incomprehensible experience. Little did I know this would be *my* experience. I can still recall a time in my life when a good friend—a physical therapist—and I were discussing the injuries of the patients with whom we had worked. We were outside having a beer while celebrating our third annual girls' weekend, a couple of months prior to my accident. At that time I was working with a few patients with brain injuries and found their challenges significant. In our discussion, my friend and I compared our thoughts and experiences. I admitted that my worst fear was acquiring and surviving a brain injury because they vary so much from one patient to another. The impairments can encompass physical, cognitive, and behavioral challenges and range from mild to severe. These factors depend on the area of the brain damaged, the severity of the injury, and the follow-up care provided.

On November 3, 2006, as I drove home from an appointment at a patient's house, my life changed. I was struck by a pickup truck on a state road. Hydraulic rescue tools (e.g., Jaws of Life) were used to extract me from my small car and save my life. I was taken by helicopter to the local hospital and underwent a craniotomy to remove a subdural hematoma. I also sustained multiple fractures on the left side of my body, which continue to affect my life today. I later developed blood clots and had to have a Greenfield filter inserted into my vena cava (large vein taking blood back into the heart) to prevent clots from entering my heart and brain.

After a few weeks in the local intensive care unit, I was taken to Bryn Mawr Rehab in Pennsylvania for 2 months of inpatient treatment. Bryn Mawr is where I woke up. This is also where my nightmare began, where I began to understand what had happened to me. I have an element of perfectionism in my personality, and to be imperfect, even if it resulted from a brain injury, was quite a challenge for me. After my accident, it wasn't uncommon for me to get people's names mixed up, like calling my boyfriend my dad or vice versa. But even with those mistakes, even with a brain injury, I knew too much from a medical standpoint. I knew that it could take a long time to recover, if I recovered. And I wouldn't have had it any other way, as this "knowing too much" helped motivate me throughout my recovery. In the beginning of my rehab, even with cognitive difficulties and memory loss, I believed that I could and would recover. I knew that I could beat this brain injury. I knew firsthand, as a therapist, the positive outcomes of rehabilitation, the neuroplasticity of the brain, and the benefits of a support system. And throughout my treatment, I worked hard and knew I would survive.

As an inpatient, I did all that I could during my therapy. This included learning and recalling my therapists' names, learning to walk using a rolling walker, and navigating other challenges. In addition to left and right hip fractures, my left clavicle and five left ribs were fractured. I had pain and limited movement, which caused my scapula to "wing." On one occasion as I reached toward the pain, I noticed that my shoulder blade was sticking out, and self-diagnosed a winging scapula. I shared that information with my boyfriend who confirmed that I was onto something. The next day I talked with my occupational therapist, and she confirmed my condition. My confidence went through the roof with my ability identify a medical condition! Now, I look back on that milestone with pride.

Following this discovery, I became more aware of the occupational therapist in me. I had the pleasure of sleeping in a bed with a zipped canopy for safety. It was difficult to watch my loved ones zip me into bed before they left me at the hospital, because I knew they hated to do that. But for my own safety, I acknowledged and accepted this. One night, however, this was especially helpful; a fellow TBI patient from down the hall escaped from his room and ended up in my room. At the time, my roommate was unable to reach her call button due to limited range of motion. She called out my name and woke me up. When she brought this "escape" to my attention, we were certainly glad that we had the zipper canopies protecting us from him. Brain injury patients can vary significantly, and sometimes they can be impulsive and resistant, which can affect the safety of others. Initially I thought the reason we were zippered in was to prevent us from escaping our own beds and wandering around. I did not realize until this night how important it was to keep others out!

After 2 months, I graduated from the inpatient facility to the outpatient day program. The daily routine of the day program felt like going to school. I had my classes, which consisted of speech, occupational, physical, and cognitive therapies, and a lunch break. When we arrived at "class" each morning, we would copy our schedules, which told us our times for therapy. Every day I worked hard to remember more and more. The use of a memory book was a great help. This consisted of my schedule of therapies, which I used to take notes about my day. In the morning, when copying my schedule, I would write the therapists' names next to my appointments. This was my morning cognitive exercise, helping me recall their names and prepare for each therapy. Following the treatment session, I would write down what I had done as a reminder. I even asked my therapists for extra cognitive activities and physical exercises to do at home on nights and weekends. As a group we would go to lunch in the cafeteria. My brain injury affected my memory and my sense of direction. In the beginning, I made sure I followed others to the cafeteria and was not the leader. As I continued with treatment, I became familiar with the hospital and mastered this problem. I lived in an apartment near the hospital for the 6 months that I attended the day program. My goal was to return to my own home, return to work, and get my life back.

I was driven to and from rehab by a transportation service. Usually one of three men would pick me up and drive me there. On one occasion, a new driver picked me up from rehab. After introducing himself, he proceeded to ask me where I lived and how to get there! Because I was recovering from a severe TBI, I had no idea how to provide him with directions. So I told him to ask someone inside from the treatment program. He did just that, but left me in the back seat of a running vehicle, parked in front of the brain injury outpatient program. When he returned to the car, I educated him about how unsafe it was to be parked in front of fellow TBI patients who may be impulsive enough to drive the car away with me in it! (Fortunately I was not impulsive enough to do so myself.)

Toward the end of my treatment, I took my driving test at the rehabilitation driving center to assess my road safety. To prepare, I practiced driving in the parking lot of a school with my boyfriend. Getting behind the wheel again was a great accomplishment, but still, it was a frightening challenge given my awareness of what driving had done to me and my life. When I was ready for my driving test at the rehab center, I got into the test vehicle with the instructor, and off we went. I was a little nervous, because it was a big step toward regaining my independence. As part of the preparations for the driving test, I had been responsible for getting directions to the destination. The instructor would direct me by reading them back to me as I drove. When we left the front of the rehab building, he directed me to a remote portion of the parking lot and asked me to park the car there briefly. I didn't think too much of it, and I did not pay too much attention to that spot; I was ready for the drive, the directions, and making sure I was a proper driver. We then departed for our drive. The drive included a variety of roads, including back roads and highway. We arrived at the destination, a car dealership, safe and sound and then went back to the rehab center. As I pulled into the large parking lot, the instructor asked me to return the vehicle to that parking spot from earlier. I circled around the building two times, and I could not find that part of the parking lot. I failed my driving test and required additional driving lessons to further assess my sense of direction and safety. With this error, I learned that I needed to pay more attention to details. This also was my first practical lesson on how much I needed to incorporate compensatory strategies into my daily life. After taking a few more driving lessons, I became more comfortable and aware. I retested and passed. When I returned home, I got a GPS to rely on for directions to both new and old destinations. Also, my return home to a familiar environment helped my sense of direction thrive.

Other compensatory strategies I used were to write everything down and use pictures to jog my memory. After 6 months of outpatient treatment, I returned to my work in outpatient rehabilitation with children. I started off with part-time hours, 3 days per week, and increased my hours every couple of weeks as I became comfortable with the expectations and duties. Building up my caseload to 8 to 10 kids per day was intense for me. It also was a challenge because all these children were new patients for me; none of them were familiar faces from before my injury. I took notes like crazy about the children and their skills during the session, making sure that I did not miss anything. I was trying to prove not only to myself but to coworkers and patients' families that I was okay. I also found it helpful to take a picture of the child to stimulate my visual system to recall activities and skills from the session when needed. I used these compensatory strategies for the first 6 months or so of my return to work.

Throughout all my rehabilitation, my role as an occupational therapist was always with me. Even though I was a patient, I was an OT. I knew the positive outcomes of therapy and the need for motivation and support that helped me with my recovery. My knowledge as an occupational therapist inspired me to be the best patient that I could be.

I have been back at work for more than 3 years now. I am proud of my friends and family who were there for me, who pushed me and encouraged me. This encouragement came from time with family and friends, phone calls, and a blog where people posted encouraging words. It was incredible to be reminded of my friends and family across the country who were rooting for me to get better, to get my life back. I am proud of my recovery, proud of "knowing too much," and proud of still being an occupational therapist even when I was a TBI patient. This experience helped me look at my life and live each and every day to its fullest. I realize that every day that I am here is a gift. We never know when our end is, we never know what life is going to throw our way, but we do have control over how we react to it. We can choose to live life on the sidelines, or we can choose to live life to its fullest.

CHAPTER 22

Practicing Who I Am: Occupational Therapy, Crohn's Disease, and Self-Management

Carol Seibert, *MS, OTR/L, FAOTA*

I used to think I had a "secret" in my occupational therapy toolbox: my own experience with the health system. I could empathize with the experience of a *patient in the health care system*. I could sympathize with complaints about hospital food and the indignity of hospital gowns. More important, as a person living with the unpredictability of a chronic disease, I knew the disorientation of being swept out of an ordinary day into an alien world of emergency rooms and diagnostic procedures.

I found that simply acknowledging the feelings my clients experienced—the uncertainty, the frustration, the hope—often established a powerful rapport. I also recognized the often unspoken expectation that going home meant getting back to normal life. However, as my home health career progressed, Crohn's disease made my own experiences as a patient more frequent and more urgent. During my first decade in home health practice, I experienced at least a dozen hospitalizations, including five surgeries, often with little warning. One day, after six home visits, I ended up in the emergency room, and by midnight I was in intensive care. I "hoarded" paid time off to ensure that I'd have an income if unanticipated surgery put me out of commission for 6 weeks or more.

My patients were seldom aware that I was concurrently their therapist and a patient, but gradually my coworkers knew. Years earlier, the disease had controlled my life. I knew too well the concerned gaze or the well-meaning comments from friends or relatives and the feeling that I was seen as a "sick person." After a life-saving surgery my senior year of college, I had no symptoms for nearly 7 years. In a different state, different work, a new career, I felt that "patient" was once again on my forehead.

I responded by finding ways to limit the impact of the disease on my work. After 9 years working full-time, I cut back to 30 hours, which still gave me access to a critical benefit: group health insurance. While my income was less, home health allowed me flexibility to control when I worked. When a new medication made it difficult for me to function in the morning, I scheduled all my visits for after 11:00 a.m. I also started looking for other professional opportunities and income that would allow me to control my schedule.

I also took charge of how people saw me as a "Crohnie." I was more vocal about having Crohn's disease. I responded to queries by soliciting donations for Crohn's disease foundation fund-raisers. Instead of "patient" I sought to project "Crohnie with attitude."

After 14 years as a home health practitioner, I parted ways with home health agencies. A community health grant turned into an opportunity to provide services similar to home health practice but with less driving and total flexibility in scheduling. This project led to a community health "chronic care" initiative. One responsibility was to co-lead the Chronic Disease Self-Management Program (CDSMP) (Stanford, 2006). The CDSMP leaders' training led me to reflect on my own experiences with Crohn's disease. During most of high school and college, Crohn's disease had ravaged my body while medications—high dose steroids—wreaked havoc with my mind and emotions.

During the CDSMP training, I came across a statement that read,

Self-Management Tasks

1. To take care of your illness (such as taking medication, exercising, going to the doctor, communicating your symptoms accurately, changing diet).

2. To carry out your normal activities (such as chores, employment, social life, etc.).

3. To manage your difficult emotional changes (changes brought about by your illness, such as anger, uncertainty about the future, changed expectations and goals, and sometimes depression, and also including changes in your relationships with family and friends) (Lorig, Sobel, Gonzalez, Laurent, & Minor, 2006).

I almost laughed out loud when I read those lines. Wasn't this what I had been doing for over 30 years? I realized there were really two stories. One story was the life I was making. The other story was the struggle to manage my disease. The two were completely intertwined.

While I had not had the term in my vocabulary previously, it seemed to me that I had been a pretty effective *self-manager* most of the time, even when my transitions from work to emergency room or surgical suite and back were pretty surreal, even to me.

Recognizing all of this forced me to reflect on my practice. I came to realize that what had also mattered was addressing the challenge my clients faced *living a life with a health condition*. I had often described my role as an OT being about *integration*. The self-management perspective—managing one's daily activities, one's health, and one's feelings—truly captured what I meant by integration.

What does this look like in my practice? Most of my clients have chronic conditions. Often their management is either/or—focusing on managing the condition and the tasks associated with this management *or* being so busy trying to deal with daily responsibilities that they don't have the time or energy for the tasks that keep their condition controlled. My practice focuses on strategies to manage specific tasks and also how to integrate or incorporate these tasks into existing daily routines. For example, teaching "energy conservation" is more than a list of "dos" and "don'ts." It's about applying a strategy—*managing energy*—and assisting my clients to apply it to their activities to do the things they need and want to do. Reframing strategies as *management*—and not "giving in" or "giving up"—is essential so that my clients recognize that the goal is for them to manage their condition instead of their condition controlling them. Being able to walk the dog, make supper for the family, or go to the mall with a teenage daughter are the things that matter to my clients—and even these simple tasks are derailed when their condition dominates their lives.

My most important realization has been that I see the impact of my practice differently. If I am truly supporting self-management, what matters most is that what I do makes a difference for the client *after* discharge. I realize how much I have appreciated providers who saw the place of their interventions in the larger picture of my life. I don't look so kindly on those who thought that what they were addressing (the disease) was the most important thing or the only thing in my life. So now I ask myself, "what difference will this intervention make for this person a month or 6 months or a year from now?" That means my job is to first to discover what "having a life" means for each client and what is associated with managing his or her condition. This is a collaboration, a dance, and it's different for every client. The common element—for myself and for my clients—is that self-management is the ultimate outcome.

References

Lorig, K., Sobel, D., Gonzalez, V., Laurent, D., & Minor, M. (2006). *Living a healthy life with chronic conditions: Self-management of heart disease, arthritis, diabetes, asthma, bronchitis, emphysema, and others.* Boulder, CO: Bull.

Stanford University. (2006). *Chronic disease self management program* [Workshops]. Palo Alto, CA: Author.

CHAPTER **23**

Two Sides of the Same Coin

Jacqueline Thrash, *OTR/L*

I have been an occupational therapist for more than 20 years and have enjoyed every minute. I have seen many cases of suffering, trauma, disability, recovery, and triumph. My most compelling story of recovery and accomplishment is one I am intimately involved with: my own.

I have been mildly disabled since the age of 10 with bilateral bunions and hammertoes. Following three foot surgeries in 10 years, I became aware that I was different and that my challenges had become a part of me. When I was 21, I moved from Virginia to California to start my life as an adult. A friend introduced me to personal care attendant (PCA) work, which helps keep adults with disabilities in their homes and communities by assisting them with activities of daily living. After working as a PCA for about a year, I sought my bachelor's degree in occupational therapy from San Jose State University. I received it in 1986 and worked in rehabilitation with individuals with orthopedic, neurological, and spinal cord injuries. I enjoyed every minute and saw both the value of occupational therapy to the client as well as the value of being a therapist myself. I learned about life, its challenges and the different ways to work it out. I learned that being human is vulnerable, and we all need help at one time or another. I was able to participate in others' journey and help them turn struggle into triumph.

Five years ago, when walking across the street in Burbank to catch the bus to work, I was struck by a van and thrown to the ground. When I landed, I felt a stabbing pain in my back and knew I had broken my spine. My head bounced off the asphalt from the momentum of being thrown backward. I said to myself, "Oh, that's not good, I could pass out from that," but I did not. I proceeded to roll out of the way so as to not be run over by the wheels. When I came to rest, the driver jumped out of the van and was freaking out from having just hit me with her van. I told her to call 911 and helped her remain calm by telling her our location when she was unable to tell the emergency dispatcher where we were. My training as a therapist assisted me in remaining calm and thinking straight in an emergency.

After 3 days in the hospital, I was sent home with a 3rd lumbar compression fracture, fractured and dislocated wrist bones, and torn wrist ligaments. The pain was awful, and my career was ruined—or so I thought. My hand and wrist were wrapped in a splint cast for 6 weeks while my insurance company tried to find a hand surgeon who would take my insurance. After my surgeon, Neil Ford Jones of UCLA, agreed to operate, we scheduled the surgery. In preparation, I consulted a hand therapist I knew to ask what I should do after surgery, and for the 13 weeks my arm was to be in a cast in order to make sure I had a good, functional hand at the end of all of this. She told me to make sure I could bend my metatarsal phalangeal joints completely and touch my thumb to all fingertips, as well as get the swelling out of my fingers and hand. I worked feverishly to get the swelling out of my fingers while I waited to heal and be ready for the cast.

Directly after surgery, I could only move my thumb a tiny bit and my index finger about half an inch. My hand was about twice its normal size, and extremely painful. I realized, though, that I could prop my hand on the mouse of my computer and click the button with my index finger, so I had a purposeful activity that I could use to improve the function of my hand. I proceeded to learn to hunt and peck with my index finger, remembering a time when I could type 75 words per minute. Oh, well, it was a beginning.

A month before my accident, I had started writing a clinical resource book about using different native languages with occupational therapy clients. I realized that now, while I was in rehab and recovering, I could write my book and use it as purposeful and meaningful activity to rehabilitate both my hand and my back through sitting for periods of time at the computer. This activity would assist me with the psychological effects of suddenly losing my occupation and could possibly ward off depression while I worked vigorously on my goal to recover and return to work.

I spent 2 years recovering, and as part of that process, I had to do everything from learning to tie my shoes again to using a can opener backward and with my nondominant hand; writing and eating for 3 months with my nondominant (left) hand, managing my pain with medication, electrical stimulation, and exercise; and building my sitting tolerance from 10 minutes to 2 hours. At first I could walk less than a block, but over several months, I worked up to 2 miles. It took a long time, and I had a lot of pain. It took me 2 months to be able to drive again, because I had a stick shift, and changing gears caused pain in my wrist. It took me 3 months to be able to get into the bathtub because of my inability to bear weight on my right wrist and my back going into spasm when I tried to sit down in the tub.

While I was recovering, I did some reflective thinking about my life, my career, and where I wanted to go from here. I realized that with hard work on my part, support from my husband, Eddie, and the services I received from several physical and occupational therapists as well as applying the principles of occupational therapy on myself, I could return to being a clinician. However, I would have to modify my work activities and consider another means of employment in the long-term because of my advancing age and residual disability.

To begin with, I realized that I couldn't go from simply being able to drive to the grocery store and back (30–45 minutes of activity) to working an 8-hour day without building up my activity tolerance. I decided that I would go to the store several times a day for a few items to build up my stamina, and when I could tolerate it, I would enroll in the local community college and take two classes a week, which amounted to 4 hours of activity a day (the bus ride there, class, and the bus ride back home) 5 days a week. At first, it was extremely taxing, and I had to bed as soon as I got home, but that was okay because I could do my homework while lying down.

I continued to build up my tolerance and kept my mind occupied by taking cultural anthropology, linguistic anthropology, voice-activated typing, interpersonal communication, introduction to linguistics, Spanish I and II, and at California State Los Angeles, a graduate level linguistics class; I also continued to work on my book. At one point, I decided that I wanted to get my master's in occupational therapy, so I began looking at different schools I could attend. I enrolled in the online postprofessional master's program at San Jose State University, my alma mater. Besides, I needed to return to work because disability payments didn't cover my bills, and I missed my career.

I finished my book in September 2006 and returned to work November 2006. My employer, interface rehab, allowed me to use an occupational therapy aide to assist with transfers and any physical activity that might aggravate my back or wrist. I was delighted to be back at work and had a renewed understanding and appreciation for the rehabilitation process, occupational therapy, and living life to its fullest.

It has been 3 years since my return to work, and 5 years since my accident. I have published the book I had worked on during recovery, *Common Phrase Translation: Spanish for English Speakers for Occupational Therapy*, and an article, "So You Have an Idea…" in *OT Practice*. I am one semester from finishing my postprofessional online master's, and my master's thesis project is to develop an in-person course to teach Spanish to occupational therapists. I completed the pilot course development, and taught the master's thesis class, "Functional Communication: Spanish for Occupational Therapists" in October 2009. Hector Borrero and I have been accepted to present a 3-hour workshop of Spanish for occupational therapy at the 2010 AOTA Annual Conference & Expo in Orlando, Florida. The highlights of the outcome of my accident is my body of work thus far, that I will be presenting a poster from my Spanish for Occupational Therapy class at the World Federation of Occupational Therapy in Santiago Chile in May 2010, and that I have been nominated for a Recognition of Achievement Award from AOTA. From all this I have experienced both sides of the same coin: being the therapist and being the patient. I have a renewed respect for therapists and patients, a renewed love of my career, a belief that all things are possible, and the satisfaction of living life to its fullest. I hope I have inspired you to do what is in you, to stretch yourself, to put your heart into your work, and to live life to its fullest.

References

Thrash, J. (2006). *Common phrase translation: Spanish for English Speakers for occupational therapy, physical therapy, and speech therapy.* Burbank, CA: Jacqueline Thrash.

Thrash, J. (2007). So, you have an idea… *OT Practice, 12*(20), 7–8.

Part V

Inspirational Clients

CHAPTER 24

Standing in the Place of Spirit

Rondalyn Whitney, *MOT, OTR/L*

My first job as an occupational therapist was in a large rehabilitation hospital. I worked in outpatient rehab, skilled nursing units, and geriatric psychiatry. I was in my late 20s, and most of my patients there were elderly. The elders I met taught me things with their eyes, their stories, and their habits. I know it might sound corny, but I felt that being gentle or kind or competent was barely a sufficient repayment of their daily gifts to me.

When I arrived at work each day, I'd check the schedule board for my patient assignments. One morning a new name, Brown, was scribbled in on my schedule. Mrs. Brown was a patient with cancer who had been admitted to the skilled nursing unit so she could receive direct care while getting yet another round of chemotherapy. That afternoon, I planned to help her sit bedside and freshen up after her long day with chemotherapy. I could gather some clinical observations about her stamina, cognition, and emotional state. What I didn't know was that an encounter with Mrs. Brown would be my first lesson in the art and spirit of therapeutic occupation. I also was sorely unprepared for the transformation that occurred when I let myself be touched by the love she had filled her life with, a life so fully lived—but I'm jumping ahead.

I expected Mrs. Brown to be frail and look infirm. Instead, she was radiant and beautiful, and her eyes were full of warmth and invitation, her face etched with the small lines that form as a result of much belly laughing. Her colorful turban dignified rather than defined the face of cancer. She spoke in lilts and pauses with a great deal of poise, and I was instantly reminded of Katherine Hepburn. Two adult children and her husband were fully engaged trying to solve a crossword puzzle; their banter was lighthearted, and the mood was cheerful. Mr. Brown was a large, attractive man, with a trimmed beard and gray hair neatly pulled back into a ponytail. He had beautiful, clear, ocean-blue eyes, a huge smile, and a face carved by a life full of contented moments. He was spirited and exuberant, had a great deal of intelligence, and was full of life. The family worked together to solve *The New York*

Times crossword puzzle, playing with the crossword clues and answers like children playing a game of kick the can.

I'm not sure I had ever before been in a room so full of life, and it imprinted itself on me, freezing in my mind like a cherished photograph. I take it out and run my mental fingers across it even today, 16 years later. Anyone could tell this family was connected by a lot of love and respect. I felt like a voyeur, an embarrassed intruder standing at the door with only a warmed towel and a washcloth. But Mrs. Brown turned and welcomed me, saying, "Oh, how thoughtful of you, dear," and pulled me into her world of love with a sparkle and a raised arm, and a barely perceptible but enormously effective "come here" flexing of her graceful fingers.

Mrs. Brown was always grateful. If I brought her an extra pillow, she'd say, "Thank you so much. That was so thoughtful. That will really help me," and made me believe I had indeed managed to discover and bring to her bed an essential act of care. Then the next day she said, "It was so great to have that extra pillow. I was able to sit up for a little bit longer—long enough to uncover another one of Will Shortz's diabolic themes embedded in the Sunday Times Crossword." I found myself walking lighter when it was time to see her, and I wanted to make her day a bit lighter in return.

Her therapeutic goal was to increase sitting tolerance. I desperately wanted this near stranger to maintain her amazing, inspirational life force. Sometimes the only thing that was appropriate was to have her sit up and sip some tea or water. Tucked inside my lab coat was her favorite tea, which I had brought from my home in the hope she could benefit from one I could offer in our afternoon sessions. I kept looking for simple ways to care for her. She eventually developed pneumonia and died.

When she died, everyone on the unit mourned. I learned about the art and spirit of therapeutic occupation: People we barely know can touch us in many different ways and sometimes very, very deeply. I hadn't read that in *Willard & Spackman*, the occupational therapy bible, and it caught me off-guard.

When Mrs. Brown died, her name went off the board, a new name went on, a new person showed up in the bed, and life seemed to go on. But I never forgot her and missed seeing her name on my daily schedule. It felt odd, somehow, to see her bed filled, and her name replaced on my clipboard. A week or two went by, and one morning her last name was on the board again: Brown. This time it was Mr. Brown,

Mrs. Brown's husband. There was no admitting diagnosis; he simply collapsed at his wife's funeral.

This man, who had been so full of life 2 weeks ago, had a chart that described him as "ashen," "sullen," and "sallow." Tests were being run, but all anyone knew was that he couldn't walk and was despondent. He wasn't eating, was in complete withdrawal, and hadn't spoken since he had collapsed. Perhaps he'd had a stroke or maybe he had he hit his head when he fell. The doctors could not measure or see anything wrong.

When I went to see Mr. Brown, he was lying in bed in a darkened room. The man in that bed was in no way similar to the man I had met when his wife was alive. Every single bit of his life was gone. He was a small man, without any life force. There was no sparkle, no exuberance—nothing but a hollow, blank stare and a man in a bed. I stood at the door with little to offer but a heavy heart. I remember thinking about being objective and employing my therapeutic self to serve as a barrier to becoming overly empathetic, but I couldn't get my mind to go any farther; it was like my mind was frozen, looking for a protocol I had misplaced.

I introduced myself. "I doubt you remember me, but I was the treating therapist for your wife." In spite of all I had been taught about professional demeanor, I started to cry. I said, "I remember her. I was so sorry when she died." Tears betrayed me more, streaming down my face. "I got to know her and you and your family during those 2 weeks she was here. I was inspired every day by her, even for the brief time I had the privilege to know her. And it really touched me to know her, and I was sorry to hear that she had died." Well, I was a very new, green professional if ever there was one, and here I stood blubbering to a man who had something much more difficult from which to recover than I did. But Mr. Brown turned and looked at me and said, "Oh, I remember you. You brought washcloths and fresh pillows and Earl Grey tea."

Therapy is about restoration of function. But what kind of goals do you set for a man who was there because his life and his wife had died together? I knew my way of interpreting his "illness" wasn't scientific, but my eyes and heart battled my scientifically trained mind. I met with my supervisor to discuss Mr. Brown's treatment and told her my feelings. I confessed that I thought his condition was more than depression and that it went beyond a physical impairment. His life had left him at that funeral. It was as if he and his wife had shared one life force. Now that life was gone, and only his body was left. I had told my supervisor about this man and his family before. Now I asked, "Pat, what am I to do?"

She said, "Look. He is at the end of his life, the life as he has lived it up to now and perhaps the end of life itself. So our main goal may be a little bit of TLC." I remembered the crosswords and the laughter with his wife during the afternoon tea he remembered sharing with me and with her. Pat said, "I trust you. Find a way to provide what's needed and keep in mind that the primary goal from the occupational therapy department is TLC for this man. Because you and I both know that he's here to die."

Each day, something new was wrong with him, and the doctors scrambled to identify or measure it. He developed bedsores seemingly overnight. A special bed was ordered. The next day he developed a rash from the new bedding and developed more skin breakdown. A new bed pad was ordered. Every day there was a new problem. This man seemed to be decaying. Both his son and daughter were searching for answers but the doctors had none.

Mr. Brown refused to eat, but I learned he loved cranberries. I had lived in Boston, so I started talking to him about the cranberry bogs on Cape Cod while handing him a warm washcloth to wipe his own face and hands. I told him how one autumn, the time of year they flood the bogs in New England, I had driven to Duxbury from Boston where, instead of the expected green fields along the road, I had seen lakes of brilliant cranberry red. The first time I saw one, there had been a fog lifting over a sea of red, and I had had no idea what it was. Mr. Brown laughed a bit at my naivete, that as an Appalachian native who had transplanted to Boston, I had been so clueless about bogs and autumn berries. He seemed to become more alert and we'd reminisce about his wife; interesting words; cranberries; and New England's idiosyncratic rituals, routines, and habits.

Although his stamina was measurably waning, he usually had a little energy for our sessions, and I was humbled that I could bring something meaningful enough to him that he would spend his sparse but precious resources with me. As I talked with Mr. Brown, I would hand him a washcloth, or I might say, "Let me help you sit up so we can visit a bit." He would sit for 20 minutes while brushing his teeth or changing his gown. But the 20 minutes became 18, then 15, and then 12.

Because he loved cranberries, I brought in some of my son's dried sweetened cranberries. I'd put them on the tray, and he'd take little pinches, kind of the way little babies nibble and play. I'd set them in little piles to his left and then to his right on the tray so he would have to reach to get them. We'd talk the whole time—about cranberries, a beautiful fall day in California, rocky beaches at Marblehead, and orange maple leaves in the autumn.

Still, Mr. Brown worsened each day. I was torn because I had learned in school that therapy was about getting better. But despite our best efforts, Mr. Brown made no progress. I was very troubled. I wasn't suppose to care this much, was I? I felt selfish for wanting him to live if he didn't want to. Who was I to want that?

One morning when I'd gone in to see him, I said, "Mr. Brown, how are you? How was your night?" He was looking at the window and said, "I saw the children dancing. They were dancing all night." He started describing children wearing halos of flowers in their hair and spring dresses, dancing and playing with hoops and running around the fountain, laughing. They were playing all night, he told me. To him they were real and made just as much sense as me standing there. He described them perfectly: He wasn't sorry they had kept him up; seeing them had really been delightful and wonderful. He looked very happy, peaceful, and calm. His curtains were completely drawn. It had been dark all night, and he was on the third floor. I knew what he was seeing because my father had reported a similar sight right before he died.

He was almost delirious now. The team began to wonder if he should be transferred to the geriatric psychiatric unit. I spoke with Pat again and told her what I was seeing and feeling. I confessed I thought this man was transitioning and the veil between this world and the other world had gotten thin. I strongly felt that this was an important experience for him to have, and he had the right to have it and *not* be transferred to a psychiatric ward. But if I was wrong, I thought Pat might escort me out of the building. "Pat, does that make me crazy? Is it possible he's just dying and telling me about it?

Pat replied, "Of course he is, Rondalyn. Take good care of him as he dies." She showed me how to call the family and coached me in what to say about his treatments and the importance of having family near him, the value of reminiscing and relationship and engagement in beloved occupations such as crosswords.

So I learned another valuable lesson as an occupational therapist: How to help a patient be restored even at the end of life.

I'm so grateful I had the kind of supervisor who valued caring for clients, who infused her wisdom with humanity to come up with a plan of care for a person and who had the courage to follow such a plan. She wasn't a religious person, and neither am I really, but we both believe in spirit and the human spirit. I was so fortunate to have a supervisor who understood my confusion and mentored me to use the full power of my profession to provide authentic care to Mr. Brown. She encouraged me to become as much of an occupational therapist as I had the heart to be. She gave me a gift once, a small note tied up in a handmade box that said, "Don't ever lose heart." I framed it with a lock of my son's hair, a seashell shaped like a wing, an orange maple leaf, and fabric the color of a cranberry bog in November. It hangs over my desk to remind me to keep my heart open.

I continued to see Mr. Brown the next couple of days. I brought in a picture of my son, and I brought in flowers from my garden. I talked about family and the importance of his family. We talked about his wife and how they spent life's moments over crosswords, took long daily walks, and enjoyed good bluegrass, rhubarb jam, Robert Frost, Johnny Walker Red, and the laughter of children. I shared how my husband and I had started working on *The New York Times* crosswords each night after getting into bed. We got visiting hours extended for his family.

I was off on Saturday and was scheduled to work Sunday. Sunday morning I had an amazing dream. It was 15 years ago, that dream, but I still remember it. Children were dancing everywhere. Mr. Brown was dancing with his wife. They were back to their blissful selves. He was talking to his family. I was on the outside watching these joyful people when Mr. Brown turned to me. He looked at me affectionately, lovingly, like a father might look at his daughter, and he kissed me very tenderly. It was a kiss like I might kiss my own son when I am most in love with him. Then he stood back, held my eye for a long time, and floated away. The dream left me full of gratitude, full of life. My first thought on waking up was how absolutely wonderful I felt. I felt like I had received a blessing.

When I got to work, I checked the schedule board as I did every day, but Mr. Brown wasn't on my list. He had died that morning.

The Browns came into my life for 4 weeks, but they changed my life forever. By knowing them, I learned my most important lesson as an occupational therapist: Spirit is something that lives in the context of a person's life, and recognizing the importance of spirit in the practice of occupational therapy is a blessing if you let it be one. A rationalist might explain what I experienced as some unsupportable, backwoods superstition. They might attribute what Mr. Brown experienced to some kind of brain misfiring. But I believe health is an important resource in life, not the reason for life. Life can be full of spirit when it is empty of everything else, and connecting with another's heart and spirit is an act of occupational engagement. Spirituality is intricately related with transcendent living and is at the heart of living life to the fullest.

I believe with all my heart that Mr. Brown came to me and kissed me to make sure I remembered his lesson. Because of Mr. and Mrs. Brown, I learned that living life to its fullest doesn't just apply to our clients; it applies to us as we authentically engage with our clients. With gratitude, I often think of the Browns who lived so well that they inspired me to do the same. I try to honor Mr. Brown's lessons to me when I teach occupational therapy students, treat new clients, parent my sons, or uncover the theme in our nightly *New York Times* crosswords.

CHAPTER 25

Natural Texan

Beth Ching, *M.Ed., OTR/L*

    I am a native Californian, but when I lived in Austin, Texas, from 1989 to 1995, I never said that too loudly. At least I was not a "Yankee" from a northern state, which would have warranted even more good-natured teasing by my native Texan colleagues. What I learned in a hurry was that Texans are by and large very proud and rooted to their state. My husband is from Laredo, Texas, but he was living in Austin when I moved there to be with him. I had been an occupational therapist for less than 5 years when I moved to Texas, and I think that is why living in Texas—at such an early point in my career—had such an impact on my formative occupational therapy development.

    I identify myself ethnically as an Asian American—more specifically as a third-generation Chinese/Korean American. I've lived most of my life in northern California, where I currently reside. Being an Asian American occupational therapist on the West Coast is not unusual. But moving to Texas was the first time I had lived outside of California, and I really did not know what to expect in terms of how I would be viewed. At that time, I knew there were not as many Asian Americans in central Texas compared to the San Francisco Bay Area. I had no idea if clients would take to me or not.

    My last occupational therapy position in Texas was at St. David's Hospital in Austin. I worked in the older adult partial hospitalization program. On one particular outing with the clients, we went to the Lyndon B. Johnson Library. Most of the older clients were able to navigate the long halls with their walkers or canes. One participant, whom I will call "Claire," seemed tired even though she walked without use of an ambulatory device. She reminded me of a Southern belle because of her demeanor, mannerisms, and elegance. She was taking a break from looking at an exhibit and was rising from the bench with some difficulty. I offered her my arm—she gave me direct eye contact and stated appreciatively, "You are the most natural Texan I ever did meet." I felt I had crossed an acceptance threshold.

Here was a native Texan paying me the ultimate compliment. But did I mention that you cannot ever claim to be a Texan unless you were born and raised there? Transplants like me did not count. I wholeheartedly accepted the verbal praise! In my humble view, this gracious White client probably never had any prolonged contact with an Asian American before, let alone a therapeutic relationship. To me, "natural Texan" translated to "you are alright!" I was being validated as a trustworthy person even though I did not share the same background or heritage as Claire.

When I was in Texas, I came to understand many lessons that guide my occupational therapy philosophy to this day: "Actions speak louder than words" is not just a cliché, Southern hospitality is alive and well, and Living Life To Its Fullest™ is a grand motto for occupational therapy. These truisms are intimately connected to each other, and I would like to explore them a bit further.

Actions speaking louder than words is integral to living life to its fullest because we are a "doing" profession. In occupational therapy, we actively assist people in meeting in their goals which they in turn put into action in their own lives. How can actions speak louder than words? I identify myself ethnically as an Asian American. When I lived in Texas, many older adults still used the term Orientals, or at least they did in the late 1980s and early 1990s when I lived in Texas. I was not bothered by this. Please do not misunderstand me; I think words have power, and language is so important. Generally, I would just point out to the client that the more current identification was Asian American. If I had to choose between the behavior of someone who spoke in politically correct terminology but treated me shabbily or someone who spoke in an outmoded fashion but treated me with respect, my preference would always be for the behavior of the person who treated me with respect. Perhaps finding more value in someone's behavior is an occupational hazard for occupational therapy practitioners, because I have had many conversations about clients who "could talk a good story but would not be able to functionally perform." So much of what we do in terms of evaluation and treatment has its basis in what people do and show through their actions rather than what they may say about what they can do.

Hospitality puts this difference between saying and doing into practice. Gracious living is a virtue in Texas, and not just at social events or parties either. If a repairman comes to my home, I should always offer him a drink of water or iced tea. Shaking hands is a general practice as opposed to just saying "hi" to acknowledge someone's presence.

When I offered Claire my arm to escort her, she did not have to take it—but she did. Hospitality is collaborative because there needs to be a sender and a receiver.

In Spanish there is a phrase, *"buen educado,"* which literally translates to "well-educated" in English. However, as I understand its common use, it really means being well-raised to treat others with courtesy and respect. Hospitality is creating an environment where people feel welcome, safe, and respected.

As I mentioned before, my husband is from Laredo, which is in southern Texas right on the Texas–Mexico border. He is Mexican American, and the Latino influence is huge in Texas, particularly in this part of the state with its proximity to Mexico. Many of the values that were infused in me from Texas have to do with what I have learned about Mexican heritage. Sure, many Americans associate Mexican culture with a party atmosphere because of the Mexican-American holiday Cinco de Mayo; however, Mexican culture is rich with tradition, complexity, and profound compassion, in my experience. Sharing time together is so precious to this culture; hence, on the surface, so many symbols for Mexican culture are simplistically depicted as partying—think tequila, margaritas, and piñatas.

In Latino culture, gatherings are a high art, a study in hospitality. Unlike English where we say, "to throw a party," in Spanish we say, *"hacer una fiesta,"* or "to make a party." Parties are not casually thrown together; parties are built from the ground up. When my husband's family has a party, everyone contributes his or her talents in some way to make a memorable event. Isn't this exactly what we do in occupational therapy? We focus on a person's strengths, and we ask the individual to contribute whatever she or he can at the time in the interest of improving the quality of the client's life so that he or she can live it to its fullest.

Speaking of parties, when making small talk at a party, many times I will be asked what I do. When introducing myself, I say what I do for a living, not what type of person I am. When a person is unable to return to his or her former work due to an accident, illness, or trauma, it can be devastating for that person's self-esteem. After I returned to Northern California, I worked with survivors of brain injuries at a community college. Most of the clients had some short-term memory loss, and it took longer for them to process new information. Their grief about their new deficits and the loss of their former roles, strengths, and self-identities was profound. Yet some pieces of their core personalities remained intact, and I appreciated how clients were able to use humor, problem-solving skills, and life experience to help their peers who were also people with brain injuries. Being in a class with other people who were survivors of brain injury helped the students overcome some of the isolation, withdrawal, and devastation that their condition had caused.

When I taught a life skills class on effective communication to prepare the students to become gainfully employed, I clearly remember one student: a single mother successfully raising four children despite having a brain injury and being unemployed at the time. As one parent of one young child myself, I felt humbled in her presence. She was taking the class in the fall semester, and it was close to Halloween. As a way to tap into long-term memories, the topic was sharing a pleasant memory about the holiday. "Pat" related that money was always scarce in her household with only one salary, but she managed to get costumes for her children when they were young. Her strategy was to buy cotton-knit pajamas of her sons' favorite superheroes and then add a mask to complete the outfits. This way the costume was not just used once but the pajamas were used throughout the year. Living life to its fullest means knowing that as a therapist, I also have the wonderful opportunity to learn from clients. As a single mother, unemployed person with a brain injury, Pat is etched in my memory because she had what many might consider barriers, but she used all of what identified her as a person into her strengths, support, and network. She taught me that embracing what may be considered challenges can lead us to strive harder to overcome barriers and help others along the way.

Living life to its fullest means "stopping to smell the roses" or taking time for reflection. Being appreciative of others giving their time, efforts, and energy is so vital to our profession. In my current position as the academic fieldwork coordinator, Level I, at Samuel Merritt University in Oakland, California, I always encourage the Fieldwork Level I students to write thank-you notes to their clinical fieldwork educators. After all, fieldwork educators are not required to take students. In my mind, fieldwork educators host students for altruistic reasons; they want to help to further our profession. This insistence on thanking fieldwork educators stems from my time in Texas, where being courteous, polite, and attentive was part of the culture. Besides, we need to do whatever we can to acknowledge our clinical fieldwork educators as much as possible.

As an assistant professor I often tell the stories of Claire and Pat to students to illustrate what it means to meet clients on their own terms so that they may live life to its fullest. Living in Texas for even a brief time was illuminating for me, allowing me to reflect on some of my core values as a person and as an occupational therapy practitioner. "Living Life To Its Fullest" means treating people with dignity and respect, which will never go out of style.

Ever since I became an occupational therapist years ago, I have observed that as a profession we like to socialize and we give great parties. Those cooking groups serve us well! We're hospitable. We create the nourishing environment in which our clients can flourish. This native Californian owes much of these values to being a Natural Texan.

CHAPTER 26

Incorporating Love in ADLs

Brian Estipona, *OTR/L*

One of the most valuable lessons I have learned as an occupational therapist that is therapy does not always involve physical exercises or daily self-care tasks. Therapy can involve a combination of physical and emotional aspects of daily life. To love another person is an activity of daily living (ADL).

Love can be expressed in many ways. It can be expressed in words and in actions. Working as an occupational therapist, I have been touched on many occasions by the beauty of being able to address the physical as well as the psychosocial aspects of illness and injury. During the early years of my career, I came across a patient who had been dealing with cancer and had a young daughter who was 3 years of age. During the initial parts of rehabilitation, this patient was too weak, fatigued, and deconditioned to even scratch her nose. We saw her daily to work on ADLs such as grooming and hygiene, established a self-exercise program with the use of therapy bands, and incorporated family training with her loving husband to help motivate her to regain her former strength. Over the course of several weeks, her strength dramatically improved. She could now raise her arms and end our sessions with a smile accompanied by two thumbs up.

From that moment on, I felt I had accomplished a lot. I helped this young woman reach an independent level with self-care and improve her quality of life. When she would get to a functioning level with one area, I would think to myself, "What can I work on now?"

One day, I realized another dimension of ADLs we sometimes forget. On that afternoon, the 3-year-old daughter came to visit for the very first time, and the visit took place during our therapy session. I had just gotten started, and the mother was still lying in bed. After consulting with another therapist, we decided to incorporate the daughter and make this visit a very meaningful session. We encouraged the patient to get up and sit on the side of the bed. I then instructed the mother to take this opportunity to give her daughter a nice heartfelt hug. From that moment, you could see the joy, the love, and the warmth the mother had for her daughter. It was a great display of strength and endurance.

Each and every one of us serves a role in life. The role of a mother or father who loves and nurtures their young is something we sometimes overlook, although it can be more meaningful than anything we teach our patients. This experience allowed me to take a closer look at patients' life roles and to know that quality of life does not always involve just self-care independence but may also involve independence to love another.

CHAPTER 27

Nathan's Eulogy

Rhoda P. Erhardt,
MS, OTR/L, FAOTA

My most memorable challenge in my 40 years as a pediatric occupational therapist was a child named Nathan. This chapter will describe how and why we met, what I learned from him during the 25
years of his short life, and the impact that he and his remarkable family
have had on my professional growth.

In writing his story, I used the *Occupational Therapy Practice
Framework* (AOTA, 2008) to organize the information in a way that
not only tells his story, but also illustrates its usefulness to today's clini-
cians. Nathan's story offers what I believe is an invaluable retrospective
case study.

Medical History

Nathan was born full-term at a weight of 8 pounds after an uncompli-
cated pregnancy, labor, and delivery. His Apgar scores were 8 and 9. His
mother, a nurse, took him to an ophthalmologist at the age of 4 months
because of his general floppiness and persistent strabismus. Recommendations were for muscle recession surgery, to be performed when he
was older. It was not until Nathan was 6 months old that a diagnosis of
hypotonic cerebral palsy was made by a pediatrician, with a subsequent
referral to a child development center for full evaluation. My role as the
occupational therapist on that team was to assess motor skills and plan
and supervise home therapy programs. However, because of scheduling
issues, Nathan was 11 months old before he was evaluated and finally
received therapy services.

Occupational Profile and Analysis
of Occupational Performance

The main concerns expressed by Nathan's parents were his significant
delays in gross motor, fine motor, and oral–motor development, which
affected almost all areas of occupation. He had no head control, very

limited hand function, and significant feeding problems. My initial evaluations revealed that not only were all Nathan's motor skills delayed, but almost all his voluntary movements were influenced by primitive reflexes, which had not been normally integrated. For example, Nathan used the asymmetrical tonic neck reflex posture to achieve eye and head stability for any functional task involving near fixation and hand use, such as reaching for a toy. This habitual pattern compromised the bilateral symmetry required for many functional tasks. Despite these limitations, he demonstrated engagement in social participation through meaningful emotional interactions with his family in occupational experiences of activities of daily living (ADLs), instrumental activities of daily living, and play.

Intervention

Most assessment and intervention models for children like Nathan use a family-centered approach combining components of developmental theory with realistic functional needs to plan therapy programs supporting health and participation in life through engagement in occupation. I had trained with Dr. Karel Bobath and Berta Bobath in London several years earlier and was optimistic that the neurodevelopmental treatment approach would be as effective for Nathan as it had been with my other clients with developmental and multiple disabilities.

In Nathan's case, my role was to create a home program that other health care professionals would ultimately carry out. My home programs, which integrate therapy principles with ADLs, usually start with weekly sessions with the family and consultations with the local occupational therapist or supervision of an appropriate paraprofessional. My sessions are then gradually reduced to twice a month, then monthly as the program becomes refined and only needs periodic modifications. However, in my efforts to create and supervise Nathan's program in his second year of life, I encountered frustrating obstacles to service delivery.

- *Obstacle 1:* Valuable time had been lost during Nathan's entire first year of life when early intervention has proved to be essential.

- *Obstacle 2:* Because their home was more than 100 miles away, the roundtrip of 200 miles was a hardship for the family to drive and not cost-effective for me to travel. Thus, we were not always able to follow the ideal frequency schedule.

- *Obstacle 3:* The family's small rural town had no occupational therapists and only one hospital-based physical therapist with no pediatric training or experience.

- *Obstacle 4:* Nathan wanted nothing to do with me! I tried to explore some handling techniques so I could teach them to the parents and other caregivers, but he cried whenever I touched him. It didn't matter if his parents were in the room or not. This frustrating experience was unusual for me as a mother of four with more than 10 years of pediatric experience.

Outcomes

I didn't give up this challenge, of course, but it was more than a year before Nathan and I became friends. During that year, Nathan began allowing a family friend to implement the home program I designed. She did her best, but progress was extremely slow. Through his preschool years and ongoing school years, he received related services, including occupational therapy, physical therapy, speech therapy, adaptive physical education, a full-time classroom aide, and mainstream experiences in the regular education classroom. I was able to consult periodically with his team and his family and perform in-depth reevaluations of hand and visual function. My general goal for Nathan during each age transition was to ensure that occupational activities reflected the entire family's goals, values, and beliefs.

In fact, Nathan never did achieve head control, independent sitting or walking, or any hand skills except switch operation. He eventually needed a feeding tube. Did that mean that he did not live his life to the fullest? Or did we help him reach his highest degree of inclusion, level of independence, and quality of life?

Table 27.1, illustrates how Nathan's team (i.e., family, professionals, paraprofessionals, friends) did everything possible to ensure that he participated in life as fully as possible. The meaning of each activity was unique—influenced by his age, life experiences, roles, interests, and situational contexts within family and community—and used therapeutically to facilitate his ability to function in daily occupations.

My favorite example of Nathan living his life to the fullest is the story of Nathan's first power wheelchair experience at 8 years of age. The technical specialist had set the motor to about 2 miles per hour. A "kill" switch was installed in case we needed to suddenly stop the chair. We put Nathan in the chair outside in a big empty parking lot. I put my

Table 27.1. Examples of Engagement in Occupation to Support Participation in Contexts

Area of Occupation	Performance Skills	Activity and Context
• Play (exploration)	• Sensory perceptual skills: Sensory events (visual, tactile, olfactory)	Touching a lamb at the zoo (community)
• Play (participation)	• Sensory perceptual skills: Sensory events (vestibular, auditory)	Sitting on mother's lap on musical merry-go-round horse (community)
• Play (exploration)	• Sensory perceptual skills: Sensory events (vestibular) • Motor and praxis skills	Floating independently on inflatable raft at a lake (community)
• ADLs (dressing)	• Motor and praxis skills (eye pointing or hand pointing)	Selecting clothes to wear (home)
• Social participation • Leisure	• Motor and praxis skills (adaptive bowling equipment)	Bowling with peers (community)
• Play (participation) • Social participation	• Motor and praxis skills (adapted magnetic Bingo wand to pick up and place game pieces)	Playing board game with neighbor peers (community)
• Education (formal participation)	• Cognitive skills • Motor and praxis skills (Big Red round pressure switch)	Operating computer (school)
• IADLs (community mobility)	• Motor and praxis skills (joystick with gated T-switch) • Cognitive skills	Operating power chair in neighborhood (community)
• Social participation	• Emotional regulation skills (display of emotions that are appropriate for the situation)	Communicating without speech his wants, needs, and happiness or unhappiness to family and friends (home and community)

hand over his and showed him all the different directions he could move the joystick. I told him that he didn't have to push very hard, to just try it and see what happened. We stepped a few feet away from him, and he began to operate the chair by himself for the first time. He went forward and backward, and even in circles, and his beautiful smile was something I'll never forget! I don't remember how long he did this, but his mother had tears in her eyes. The joy on his face was just like every other child experiencing those first baby steps or the first time riding a bike. For the first time in his life, Nathan was moving through space all by himself!

It wasn't until Nathan was 13 years old that magnetic resonance imaging (MRI) technology discovered that he had been misdiagnosed with cerebral palsy. His true diagnosis was a rare form of leukodystrophy, a degenerative condition characterized by atrophy of the cerebral white matter and cerebellum with mental capacity relatively preserved. His parents were told that he had only a few years left to live and would face gradual deterioration of brain white matter, resulting in blindness, deafness, cognitive loss, coma, and eventually death.

However, Nathan lived for 12 more years, maintaining all mental and physical functions except pulmonary endurance. Because of frequent respiratory struggles and the loss of 70% of lung capacity, Nathan needed to be schooled at home, but he graduated with his high school class.

Nathan died at 25 years of age with his awareness, humor, and smile intact. One year later, because of genetic concerns for their other son, Nathan's parents met with an international group of physicians for an individual case consultation at a conference of the United Leukodystrophy Foundation. After studying all Nathan's medical records and MRIs, they finally decided on a more exact leukodystrophy diagnosis: hypomyelination atrophy of the basal ganglia of the cerebellum. Only 20 cases then existed in the world, and none appeared to have genetic implications.

What has Nathan meant to me and to many others? I learned so much from him. I learned that although he couldn't walk or talk, he was very good at communicating his needs, and he loved and enjoyed his family and friends. I also learned what special kinds of problems he had making his body work and what kind of therapy helped and what did not. This valuable information is what I put in a book and video that I have used to teach therapists, teachers, nurses, school psychologists, eye doctors, and many others (Erhardt, 1989, 1990).

Nathan has had a huge impact on people he didn't even know. Since the book was published (when Nathan was 10 years old), he has helped me teach professionals and parents in 29 cities in 19 states in the United States, three cities in Canada, three in Australia, and in Argentina, Finland, and the Netherlands. That's 38 presentations at workshops and conferences in more than 15 years, with an average number of 50 people attending, sometimes up to 200. That means that a minimum of 2,000 people have learned from Nathan! If we realize that most of these professionals have a caseload of 20 to 40 children at any given time, the number of children with disabilities who may have been helped by Nathan is somewhere between 40,000 and 80,000! This does not include all the university programs and clinics that bought the book and video for teaching purposes. To tell the truth, when I started compiling these numbers, I did not expect them to be so high, and it doesn't stop. By teaching my vision course online for AOTA (Erhardt, 2006), I can continue to share Nathan's story with more practitioners in this country and all over the world.

As impressive as that may be, there's a more basic reason that I know Nathan's life of 25 years was important and that he lived his life to its fullest. It's the same reason that I value the lives of all the children with disabilities who have taught me what I need to know. Nathan had a great deal of love to give, and he learned how to do that from all the people that loved him. I believe that the measure of all our lives is about the love that we give and receive.

Nathan has been and will continue to be a significant person in my life. I will most of all remember his sweetness and his humor.

References

American Occupational Therapy Association. (2008). Occupational therapy practice framework: Domain and process (2nd ed.). *American Journal of Occupational Therapy, 62,* 625–688.

Erhardt, R. P. (1989). *Administration of the Erhardt Developmental Vision Assessment.* Maplewood, MN: Erhardt Developmental Products.

Erhardt, R. P. (1990). *Developmental visual dysfunction: Models for assessment and management.* Maplewood, MN: Erhardt Developmental Products.

Erhardt, R. P. (2006). *Motor components of vision in children with disabilities.* Retrieved July 4, 2009, from http://www.dynamic-online.com

Part VI

Client's View

CHAPTER 28

Occupational Therapy for All

Jill S. Harris

There they are, clear as day: two miniature human beings scuba diving inside my body. Twelve weeks old. They are the reason I had been enjoying "enhanced" symptoms of pregnancy: double the nausea, double the growth of body parts above and below the navel. As I looked at the ultrasound picture, it almost appeared as though the divers waved at me. Arms and legs were moving, blood was pulsing, hearts were beating. Cool.

Turning my head to look at my husband, I saw his nervous smile trying to convey confidence. It showed a little bit of fear. This was the third time we had been here. "It looks like twins," the doctor said this time. Twins. But 3 years earlier, the first time I had lain here for the same reason, the ultrasound did not verify life. Instead, it confirmed that there had been two lives, but they were over almost before they had begun. That day had not been about fear. It had been about sorrow.

Since then, our daughter McKenna's birth 1 year later had been normal, and she was now approaching 3 years of age. I was healthy, and we were ready to expand our family. This time the discovery that there were two just seemed vaguely familiar. We both hoped these little guys would arrive as planned.

They did.

From the very beginning, the two boys were different. That's no surprise—even mothers of identical twins will say the same thing. But the differences between them went beyond physical features and personality. It was as if they had two radically different ways of engaging the world. Baby "A," named Campbell, was immediately alive, awake, alert, and enthusiastic. Baby "B," named Wylie, almost always seemed like he had something on his mind—like he was thinking about the number pi or considering quantum physics. He ate, slept, and responded like a normal baby at the milestone appointments. There was just always something unique about him.

My mom was the first to comment that Wylie seemed to always hum. When he slept he made noises. When he was awake, he seemed to make noises more than Campbell. At about 3 months of age, Wylie found his middle two fingers, and they were almost constantly in his mouth, especially when he needed comfort. Neither one of the boys took a pacifier, but Wylie needed his fingers. When he was a toddler, we used to joke that Wylie was "smoking" them: He would remove his fingers only to speak or comment on something. Truly, he was addicted! And just like smokers sometimes take their nicotine with coffee, Wylie took his fingers with a blanket (Figures 28.1 and 28.2).

Child psychologists teach and most parents are aware that children have favorite blankets and toys. This is not unusual. However, Wylie's preoccupation with fingers and blankets was the first sign of needs that went beyond comfort and security. Wylie's preoccupations were coping mechanisms necessary for him to survive the 14 hours per day that he was awake. Fingers and blankets would later turn into laces properly tied and food groups carefully parsed, into ears covered during toilet flushes, into schedules carefully planned and consistently executed, into haircuts given with extraordinary care, into peanut butter

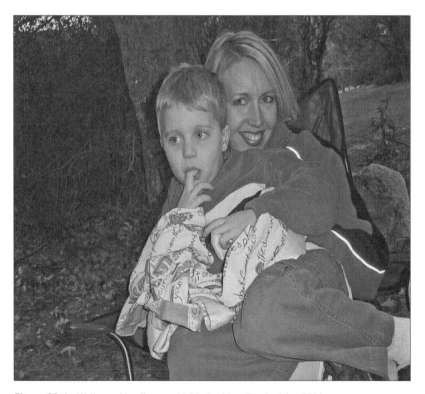

Figure 28.1. Wylie smoking fingers with blanket blue, Thanksgiving 2001.

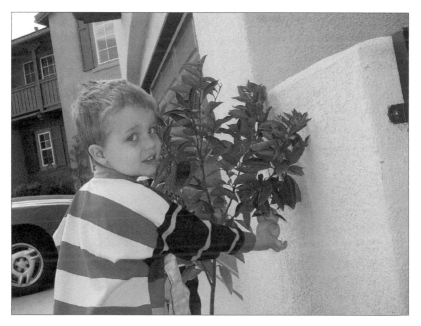

Figure 28.2. Notice how the fingers are extended? He was always careful not to touch anything else with them.

and jelly sandwiches made with precise specifications, into preschool teachers lovingly making exceptions, and into speech–language pathologists and school psychologists gingerly delivering the news to us: Wylie is undeniably and diagnostically *different*.

Wylie's experiences with occupational therapy began after his initial diagnosis as at risk for Asperger's syndrome in the spring of 2003. Weekly occupational therapy visits at the Sensory Center became a part of our lives when Wylie started school in a county program.

From day one, Wylie loved the room filled with really cool toys, scooters, balls, balance beams, zip lines, swings, trampolines, games, a ball pit, and bean bags! He eagerly anticipated every appointment to "play."

Over the course of Wylie's 6 years in occupational therapy, he was treated by various practitioners. There was work to do! An analysis showed that Wylie had a deficit in 12 of the 16 sensorimotor components, with the greatest deficits in equilibrium/protective reactions (45%), vestibular processing (38%), antigravity flexion (34%), motor planning (32%), and visual processing (29%). An assessment of his motor proficiency revealed Wylie was in the 3rd percentile for his age for fine motor skills, and he was unable to complete subtests for upper-limb coordination and balance.

Intervention for Wylie focused on two components: (1) vestibular processing as a foundation for visual–motor control and (2) proprioceptive and tactile processing as a foundation for fine motor skills. I remember reading these words and thinking, "Is there a language called "OT-speak" that I am unfamiliar with, or do these phrases have dual meanings?" With a little bit of conversation, I came to understand that the occupational therapist had found evidence of what I had observed throughout Wylie's development: He did not seem in command of his body.

I will admit that at the beginning of our occupational therapy adventure I was not a true believer in it. The way services were structured in our district, I had to provide transportation for Wylie from our school to the Sensory Center every week. This constituted a one-way trip of 20 minutes with no traffic. So on some days we spent more time in the car getting to and from therapy than Wylie received in therapy! My doubt was compounded by the fact that each visit meant Wylie missed valuable class time at school. The progress in his first couple of years was slow and sometimes nonexistent. At one point, there was also considerable turnover in the staffing of the Sensory Center, which did not improve my confidence in occupational therapy

In spite of these initial obstacles, over the years we began to see improvement in Wylie's fine and gross motor skills as a direct result of therapy. He started to cut along a straight line with scissors, write with much improved control (although penmanship is still a weak area), maintain balance, and cross over midline to play catch. Wylie's core muscle strength improved, and he learned to cope with some of his more extreme sensory issues—those involving taste, smell, and tactile areas.

In 2006, all the Harris children began age-group swim lessons. The addition of swimming into Wylie's routine really enhanced his occupational therapy efforts. His team commented on his improved performance, and they all were excited about the progress Wylie began to make after swimming for just a few months.

Although my enthusiasm for our weekly visits might have been lackluster, Wylie's excitement more than made up for my doubt. He loved occupational therapy! If the school schedule was such that a holiday took us out of a therapy session, Wylie literally cried. He befriended every occupational therapist assigned to him and learned to beautifully navigate change when a new therapist began working with him. His strong desire to please and his work ethic impressed every professional who crossed his path.

Occupational therapy provided continuity in assessing Wylie's overall development. His traditional school teachers changed every year, and each one faced a significant learning curve as he or she got to know Wylie and adapted to his special needs. The occupational therapists transcended the classroom environment and provided invaluable insights designing Wylie's overall learning goals and objectives. It may seem improbable that 45 minutes per week 30 weeks per year could yield such keen insight, but this once-skeptical parent can vouch for the results.

Before Wylie "graduated" from occupational therapy in the spring of 2009, he had not only met every one of his goals and objectives, but he had blossomed into a young man who helped other children at the Sensory Center. Each of his deficiencies had been carefully exercised into proficiency. Through this 6-year adventure, his social behaviors had also developed, transforming Wylie from a shy, young kindergarten boy who was overwhelmed by sensory experiences into a strong, outgoing fifth grader who embraced new challenges of all kinds—even a zip line over a 300-foot ravine at summer camp! How gratifying it was for our occupational therapy friends to see Wylie leave the center! His transformation was remarkable.

Wylie's occupational therapy experiences spilled over to our family, too. Tips and techniques I learned from years of observing Wylie (and reading suggested materials from our center), like "heavy jobs," helped my other children at home to organize themselves. For example, playing tug-of-war with our bed sheets at night became an evening ritual that not only got the beds prepared for sleep but prepared the kids to rest and relax. Games for the family or for play with other children at our home almost always involved fine and gross motor skill practice.

Not every child with Asperger's syndrome struggles with motor skills issues like Wylie, but it appears that most like Wylie do have sensory issues. For example, things like throwing and catching a ball, walking across a balance beam, swinging a bat, jumping up and down on one foot, descending stairs, using scissors, jumping rope, and doing other regular physical activities can be difficult for children with Asperger's. These normal—some would even say trivial—activities are not unimportant! The connection between motor skill development and academic performance and emotional behavior is well documented.

From occupational therapy practitioners I learned how to engage Wylie in physical sensory activities that supplemented his normal routine at school. These activities facilitated readiness to sit still, pay attention, write, compute, or do whatever else might be necessary in the classroom. My stories and Wylie's obvious improvement have often caused other parents to inquire if their child (or husband) could attend occupational therapy!

From what I have observed of this wonderful group of amazing professionals, I believe there is not a person on the planet who would not benefit from some form of occupational therapy. In these times of shrinking budgets and difficult economic choices, it is imperative that essential services like occupational therapy remain available to and accessible by those needing them! Maybe we should write our congressmen and congresswomen and allocate some of our tax dollars to underwrite a Sensory Center in Washington, DC—just outside the Capitol. That way, before members of Congress meet to vote on legislation and other matters affecting us, they can all participate in some good old-fashioned therapy to get "organized" and better pay attention to the tasks at hand!

CHAPTER 29

Discovering Myself Through Occupational Therapy

Sam Smith

After two job losses, I knew something was wrong. It was the mid-1990s, and I was without work in Washington, DC, a city where I had no friends or support network. I knew my disability had finally caught up with me, but I didn't know much about it. My quest to discover more about my disability led me to occupational therapy and to righting my life.

I first realized something was wrong when I was a kid in New York City in the early 1960s. I was uncoordinated and had problems learning. Basic things like tying my shoes and knowing the difference between left and right were difficult. I even had to drop out of Cub Scouts because I couldn't tie a knot. Playing musical instruments was out of the question because I had problems following the notes. I was excluded from sports by my peers because I was so clumsy. But what I lacked in motor and perceptual skills I made up by learning about social studies and reading. By the sixth grade I was reading *The New York Times* from cover to cover.

As I got older, after much questioning on my part, my parents finally shared with me that I had suffered a lack of oxygen at birth that could have led to minimal brain damage. This is apparently what psychological tests had concluded when I was a child. However, my parents did not want to stigmatize me, so I stayed in regular classes even though it was a struggle for me. Somehow I got by.

To compensate for my fine motor challenges, I wore shoes without laces. When a necktie was called for, and I didn't know how to tie a tie, I simply refused to wear one. Since I couldn't tell the difference between my right and left shoes, I put them on by feel and trial and error. Luckily for me, there weren't many tests assessing if I could tell left from right once I reached adulthood.

In college I succeeded because I could make choices about the courses I took. I knew I could do well in courses such as politics, social studies, psychology, and sociology, so that is what I took. Along the way I got interested in journalism and starting working for the college newspaper and radio station. Journalism tied together several of my interests: my curiosity about the world and my love for government and politics. I had found my passion. Again my challenges reared their head, in the form of language processing.

My language-processing deficits meant that writing clean, error-free copy, particularly on a deadline, was sometimes a daunting task. Fortunately for me, my first jobs allowed me to write and then have editors clean up my copy. But with the increased use of computers this luxury began disappearing. By the time I arrived in Washington, journalists were expected to write and report and rely less on editors to clean up copy, which ultimately led to my unemployment. My challenges were preventing me from truly engaging in my passion—writing. Faced with depression, I turned to a psychologist who urged me to fully define what my challenges were. I decided to take neuropsychological testing to learn more about my disability. There I was in my late 30s taking neuropsychological testing. Little did I know the extent of my issues! I finally understood why I had so many problems that just didn't go away. The neuropsychologist said I had more than just minimal brain damage, I had global hemispheric disorder. This disorder affected all areas of my life. I had the visual–spatial level of a 5-year-old and had severe problems with fine motor coordination, balance, processing, organization, planning, social interaction, and the ability to identify my fingers. The neuropsychologist was amazed that I had even gone to college and held a professional job. There I was, wanting to get on with my life and being told I shouldn't have even been able to do what I had done.

I don't remember who exactly told me about the Washington Developmental Center, an occupational therapy clinic in Silver Spring, Maryland. There, an occupational therapist built on the neuropsychological testing and revealed additional problems with sensory defensiveness. This explained my inability to wear jeans, put hairspray in my hair, or apply lotion to my body.

Now I was ready to work on my problems using occupational therapy. The clinic looked like a gymnasium with a ball pit, trampoline, and apparatus swings. I would be the only adult attending a clinic that looked more like a playground than anything else. A few days later I would find myself on these apparatuses working on various activities involving balance, coordination, and core body strength. The exercises helped improve my balance and coordination. Visual–spatial activities, such as putting together block patterns, and other visual activities helped me organize what I saw. Although I was only able to receive services for a few months at the center before a job opportunity in New Jersey came my way, my positive experiences propelled me to seek out a new occupational therapist when I moved.

My new clinic was called the Jeanetta Burpee Center and advocated an aggressive approach to my problems, including applying a small brush over my skin to help decrease my sensitization problems, using Swiss balls to improve balance, and attending the gym to improve my low muscle tone. My therapist even took me to her gym to do weight training. My OT also worked on activities of daily living, including learning how to floss my teeth and improving my shaving technique.

It was a visit to my home from my occupational therapist that led to a whole new realm of therapy. I had just moved to a new apartment in Philadelphia, and my occupational therapist, Beth, had come over to help me get my new apartment in order. What she found led to the beginning of a new program to help me at home and in the community. All over my apartment Beth saw torn empty boxes. It was the aftermath of my move. Instead of breaking down the boxes in a matter of minutes, I had spent hours trying to tear them apart. My apartment was filled with torn box pieces. Beth showed me the better technique that took minutes. She also realized that I needed intense help to live in my apartment independently.

I didn't know how to cook or keep my apartment in order, so my therapist came up with the idea of recruiting graduate occupational therapy students to act as life-skills counselors to assist me at home and in the community. My first student, Karen, helped me with organization and cooking. I figured I would know everything I needed to know about life within 12 weeks, which coincided with her graduation. What I didn't understand then was that my problems couldn't be easily fixed and that ongoing intervention would be needed to allow me to live at the highest level possible. I would be dealing with these problems to some degree for the rest of my life.

But that's not to say that life couldn't get better and that I wouldn't have the joy of learning new things each and every day. One of my problems, I discovered, was that I couldn't ask for help with things I didn't know were issues. If I took the lid off the cup of coffee to drink it, it wasn't because I liked taking off lids; I didn't realize there was a small hole in the cap to help drink the coffee with the cap on. Or if I ate the ice cream from an ice cream cone as opposed to licking it, it was because my tongue didn't have the range to lick the ice cream, which I didn't realize. I just assumed everyone ate ice cream that way.

The occupational therapy students acting as my life-skills counselors discovered these issues that I would have never known about. The coffee cup issue was easily resolved, but licking ice cream is a skill I am still working on.

The good news is that OT has helped me with many things—most important, remaining independent. My balance and coordination have improved, and I have fewer falls and spills. Other things are still a work in progress, such as some visual–spatial issues.

Employment is also an issue, as I recently lost my job again. I have actually improved my job skills over the years, particularly my writing, but the Internet has put a premium on quick writing and having copy perfect in a matter of seconds.

As I look back on the impact of occupational therapy on my life, I realize that without it I could not have engaged fully in living and—even more important—owning my life. A psychologist may look at how a person thinks and a physical therapist may focus on how a person moves, but the occupational therapist helps a person put everything together and own it. They help put the living into a person's life. Not so long ago I was struggling with the challenge of wearing a seat belt in the car. I have always hated wearing one. A psychologist tried to interpret my resistance, but I couldn't quite figure out why I was resistant. The occupational therapist helped me realize that my sensory defensiveness was the issue and helped me find a way to cope with the problem. I am now safe in my car.

I recently moved to South Florida, and thanks to some helpful occupational therapy faculty members at Nova Southeastern University and Florida International University, I have a new group of students teaching and helping me as life-skills counselors. I am learning how to swim. I even went kayaking, and to my amazement I was able to balance the boat and not tip over. These are things I would not have attempted several years ago. Today I put on a scuba mask for the first time in my life and went snorkeling in a swimming pool. Soon, it might be in the ocean, and for the first time in my life, I am thinking that scuba diving may be in my future.

What other professional besides an occupational therapist would take you to an amusement park as part of therapy and use a roller coaster to improve your vestibular system tolerance level? One of my occupational therapists in Florida, Amy Perry, did just that. I shudder to think what she has planned next, but then again creativity is a hallmark of the occupational therapy profession. I don't know what it would be like to live life without a disability because I have had problems from birth. But if I didn't have a disability, I would have never discovered occupational therapy and met some of the most wonderful, amazing people in the world. The encouragement and support I have received has been remarkable. With occupational therapists on my team, the possibilities are endless!

The author wishes to thank Judith Parker, chair of the Occupational Therapy Department at Nova Southeastern University, for her inspiration, her positive support, and contributions to this article. He would also like thank Nova Southeastern occupational therapy graduate student Shawna Snow for her mentorship and support.

CHAPTER 30

"I Want an OT": How Occupational Therapy Almost Missed Helping Me Live Life to Its Fullest

Chris Davis

I had called in "exhausted" on Thursday, which was to have been my first day back in the American Occupational Therapy Association (AOTA) office in Bethesda, Maryland, catching up after traveling to the Annual Conference & Expo in Long Beach in May 2005. Because California is my favorite place to visit, my husband came out for a few days after the conference, and we rented a Mustang convertible to race in style down Pacific Coast Highway to San Diego and Coronado Island for 2 days. As director of AOTA Press, the preparations for the conference had been particularly stressful; even after a few days' vacation I was unable to get out of bed until noon. Spending an unusually gray Friday in May trying to remember and document everyone I had talked to at Conference and what we had talked about to follow up for book acquisitions was draining. While in the office I thought, "A quiet weekend will change my outlook."

I was distracted all afternoon, having developed a headache early in the day that several doses of pain medication did not resolve. In the long commute home over two mountains in a thunderstorm, I became nauseated in the stop-and-go traffic with the stifling defroster on, but thankfully, my husband, my usual commuting partner, was driving my beloved Thunderbird roadster so I could close my eyes. I tried to get my mind off feeling bad by calling a friend and catching up. While sitting in the idling car at the local doughnut shop, I lost all feeling in my right hand and dropped the cell phone. As my husband jumped back in the car with his weekend supply of junk food, he noticed that I was slurring my words. He asked if I remembered where the hospital was, as we had just moved to an unfamiliar rural county only a month before. I shook my head "no" and tried to point in the general direction. My right arm would not move. What I had been slowly realizing but firmly trying to ignore during the past few hours finally had become a reality—I was 39, and I was having a stroke.

A call to 911 by my husband yielded directions from our location at Krumpe's Donuts in Hagerstown, Maryland, to the Washington County Hospital just a few miles away and had medical personnel waiting at the curb with a wheelchair. I was determined to get out of the car under my own power and clumsily pushed aside the nurses trying to help me. I stumbled into the chair, clutching my purse, fumbling for my insurance card in my disorganized wallet, and trying to instruct my husband with some authority to park "my baby" someplace safe. Once inside, the neurologist on call asked for my permission to shoot me with something to break up a suspected blood clot (a recombinant tissue plasminogen activator, or tPA, which could have side effects of additional brain damage and severe bleeding), as well as to transport me by helicopter in severe weather back to Bethesda to a better-equipped hospital near AOTA for treatment (today, my local hospital has a newly accredited stroke center). I nodded yes but became agitated thinking that one or both of those requests was ultimately going to kill me.

Then the symptoms stopped abruptly, except for a temporary but disagreeable personality change and occasional outbursts about wanting to go home, which I learned later are normal reactions to brain damage, so no need for that injection. Severe lightning had grounded the helicopter. It was dusk when I was admitted, I fell into a deep sleep in the emergency room, and at midnight I woke up in the intensive care unit (ICU). I remember, albeit vaguely, my first words to the nurse after I located my pale and worried husband leaning on the foot of the bed: "I want an OT. Really!"

To do my job well, I rely heavily on having a highly functioning brain as well as a great deal of stamina and patience. My family, which includes my husband and my elderly grandparents who practically raised me, depends on me having a reasonably well-paying job to support our household—and this work has contributed to our move from generations of poverty solidly into the middle class (no pressure!). I had been working at AOTA for 3 years and knew enough to understand that by the time I had dropped the phone in my lap, I should have been on my way to the emergency room—but I did not want to face what might be happening to me. Yet I was certain when I woke up that if I was going to be able to live *my* life to its fullest, I needed occupational therapy.

My original and subsequent requests in the ICU were met with puzzled looks, as if no one realized that occupational therapy could assist with my inability to remember events and sequence tasks correctly, my newly illegible handwriting, some driving difficulties, and the un-remitting fatigue that followed in the first few months after the stroke (my OT colleagues at AOTA correct me by calling it a *transichemic attack*, but it was scary, so I will continue calling it a *stroke*). Sure, I was very lucky not to have experienced severe functional deficits such as full and lasting paralysis, loss of vision (I read for a living!) or speaking ability, and massive brain damage. If only because of the grace of God and my husband's quick thinking, I fared far better than most stroke survivors (see Sabari & Lieberman, 2008, p. 7, for some statistics about the in-cidence and severity of stroke), but I needed to get closer to what was normal for *me* to make everything that my family had worked toward a reality. Add to that the fact that I define myself almost solely by my work and it might be easy to understand why I became insistent on receiving occupational therapy.

After getting the medical staff to send me home less than 48 hours after I had arrived so I could get some rest in my own bed and plan the week's worth of sometimes uncomfortable testing (and also call AOTA and tell them what had happened), I began to worry. Would I be able to return to work with nearly 2 decades of accumulated (and hard-won) publishing knowledge and top-flight editing skills still in my head? Would my newly hired supervisor think I could do a job with such a heavy workload while I was going through rehabilitation for "invisible" disabilities? If not, would my family lose that 1907 Tudor/Craftsman on the hill in a safe, clean neighborhood that we had saved for decades to buy? Would my husband be able to take care of me without losing his job and ultimately our health insurance? Would a baseball team's worth of nieces and nephews who love and rely on me now be scared of the new, "grumpy" Aunt Chris?

A few days later as I struggled to keep down the tiny camera on a string that I was swallowing to take a picture of my heart, I tried to mentally work out a plan for moving forward with getting better. As I was falling asleep from the anesthesia required for the test, I wondered, "What if I had not worked at AOTA when I had my stroke and had not known that I needed occupational therapy?"

What if indeed! Having the job that I do allows me to read nearly everything AOTA Press/AOTA publishes about occupational therapy (I have years of psychology, nursing, and other medical publish-ing experience as well), so I am somewhat better informed than most health care consumers. I have been engaged with the many important occupational therapy issues being debated today, which are also some of the same ones debated nearly a century earlier, sometimes without an ultimate resolution and sometimes with the discussion coming right back to where it started (e.g., scope of practice, autonomy, philosophy, specialization). Although this literature has yielded some thought-provoking and valuable ideas, it would seem that the profession now needs to invest some time and resources toward resolving some of the more "practical" issues on its to-do list—like getting the word out about this (quality of) life-saving profession to other health care professionals and potential clients. "The value system which underlies our therapeutic practice with... clients is often in conflict with our values regarding what the...profession ought to do...to have a greater impact on society" (Yerxa, 1979, as cited in Reed & Peters, 2008).

Surely the visibility of occupational therapy has been and continues to be a cause for concern. AOTA highlighted the issue in its *Centennial Vision* (AOTA, 2007) by expressing a desire for the profession by 2017 to be "a powerful, *widely recognized,* [italics added] science-driven, and evidence-based profession with a globally connected and diverse workforce meeting society's occupational needs" (p. 613). But, that I have had to push—sometimes unsuccessfully—for occupational therapy services, not only for me but for members of my family, tells me that there is much more work to be done. At my local hospital, there were surely occupational therapists and occupational therapy assistants, but they were concentrated in home care for physical rehabilitation with, for example, patients who had fallen and broken a hip (I met several when my grandfather fell on the ice a few years later). For issues that affect cognition and more complex instrumental activities of daily living—and activities that I personally might consider purposeful or my occupational choice—I was pretty much on my own.

Later at AOTA I attended a 2-day meeting of the profession's leaders and thinkers to develop the *Centennial Vision.* During the course of a conversation on descriptors about the profession, the word *power* was tossed out as an aspiration. Half the room recoiled in horror, audibly gasping at the mere mention of the word. I remember being surprised at this reaction: "Really?! Your clients *need* OT to be powerful," I thought. Mind you, it is not the power that comes from capriciously imposing your will on someone, which is what I suspect was behind the groans of the mostly female audience, but the power that comes from strength of knowledge and a respected, visible position.

If not for occupational therapy, I would not be living life to its fullest. With some accommodations, I returned to work 2 weeks later (my stroke was caused by the effects of hormone-replacement therapy and not cardiac or hematology issues), continuing to build, alongside understanding and very capable colleagues, a high-quality scholarly publishing program—and doing my part to highlight the value of the profession. My family currently has a firm hold on our hard-won financial security, and I am still a most favorite and fun aunt. All these things matter to me a great deal. For that I am eternally grateful and will remain the one of profession's biggest evangelists.

However, I want occupational therapy to be there for me when I am 80 as well. To do that, the profession's services must be easier to find and to fund. I want to walk into the local aging-in-place center housed in my neighborhood hardware store and have an occupational therapy–contractor team come to my home and help me make appropriate changes to be able to age in place. I want an OT to help me be able to navigate those ever-shrinking communications devices so I can stay connected (where are the OTs at Apple and Research in Motion who should be helping make the iPhone and Blackberry more accessible?). I want an OT to help my husband continue to be able to ride a bike or something similarly enjoyable for outdoor exercise, as well as be able to play his guitar. I want my nieces and nephews—both those on the autism spectrum and those not—to overcome various disabilities and gain a good education and careers that allow them to keep our family moving toward realizing the American dream. All of these things will help me continue to live my life to its fullest.

To make this happen, occupational therapy will need to take AOTA's Living Life To Its Fullest™ brand to heart and run with it (check out "Be a Champion for Occupational Therapy" at www.aota. org). Maybe that means you become more entrepreneurial or are one of the first to travel a new avenue for practice—and communicate your successes and challenges along the way. Perhaps that means you do research in a long-ignored practice area to "prove" that occupational therapy is effective and thus necessary. You might have to walk into the office of your local, state, or national elected officials, introduce yourself, and explain succinctly but proudly how you can help resolve complex issues of, for example, meaningful, high-quality employment for the forthcoming generation of young adults with autism; the appropriate public safety response to the country's growing cases of dementia; or even health care reform. But don't take my word for it. In Carolyn Baum's (2007) Farewell Presidential Address, she prefaces a comparable to-do list for the profession with what I have been trying to say in these pages: "Everyone you serve is counting on you to help them do what they want and need to do" (p. 620). Really!

References

American Occupational Therapy Association. (2007). AOTA's *Centennial Vision* and executive summary. *American Journal of Occupational Therapy, 61,* 613–614.

Baum, C. M. (2007). Achieving our potential [Farewell Presidential Address, 2007]. *American Journal of Occupational Therapy, 61,* 615–621.

Reed, K. L., & Peters, C. O. (2008, October 6). A time of professional identity, 1970–1985—Would the real therapist please stand up? [Occupational Therapy Values and Beliefs: Part IV]. *OT Practice,* pp. 15–18.

Sabari, J., & Lieberman, D. (2008). *Occupational therapy practice guidelines for adults with stroke.* Bethesda, MD: AOTA Press.

Part VII

New Pathways

CHAPTER 31

In the Service of Children and Families: The Making of an Advocate

Leslie L. Jackson, *MEd, OT, FAOTA*

> **Advocacy:** *ad·vo·ca·cy (noun): the action of advocating, pleading for, or supporting a cause or proposal* (Merriam-Webster's Dictionary of Law, n.d.).

> **Advocate:** *ad·vo·cate (verb): to speak or write in favor of; support or urge by argument; recommend publicly. (Noun): a person who speaks or writes in support or defense of a person, cause, etc., or pleads for or in behalf of another; intercessor* (Dictionary.com Unabridged, n.d.).

Sometimes it's hard to believe that I've been an occupational therapist for nearly 30 years. As I reflect on my career, I realize now that I have always been an advocate for the profession, always promoting some aspect of occupational therapy to educators, parents, administrators, members of my family, and students. Relatively early in my occupational therapy career, I knew I wanted to do something to improve the way children's and families' needs were or were not being met. It took some time for me to figure out all the pieces that needed to be in place and to recognize the role that policy played. This is the story of that journey.

It is no accident that my work as an occupational therapist has been with children and their families. I've been advocating for children most of my life, even before I knew what that word meant, whether by being a "big sister" to my siblings' friends, spending many hours on the front porch "counseling" them or being a sounding board for whatever was on their minds; or by pushing for respect for single parents from the social services agencies, schools, and doctors offices I had to interact with for my own children; or by recommending school-based or early intervention occupational therapy services for the children I've worked with.

My Beginning as an Occupational Therapy Advocate

My life as an occupational therapist did, however, begin by accident. I stumbled across the profession as I was preparing for a high school health class assignment my senior year. At the time, I wanted to do one of two things: play professionally in an orchestra or concert band (I play percussion) or help people. I was a little vague on the specifics of what I meant by help people, but I knew I did not want to be a doctor or nurse. I remembered that my mother had had physical therapy after her mastectomy in the early 1970s, and I always wondered what else they could have done other than having Momma squeeze a rubber ball and walk her fingers up the wall.

So I was looking through our *World Book Encyclopedia* (I am probably really dating myself here!) and came across a description of physical therapy. There, at the end of it, was the phrase: "See also Occupational Therapy." Not having any idea what occupational therapy was, I looked it up in the encyclopedia and read the description. I don't remember what it said, but it was enough to get my attention. I was intrigued and thought, "I could do that!"

I started college as a music major but decided after my son was born that I really needed a more stable career with a steady paycheck. One day, I was looking through the course catalog and saw preoccupational therapy listed as a major. Although I still didn't know any more about occupational therapy than I did in high school, I decided to change my major. I have never regretted that decision and haven't looked back since.

My son's birth was a significant event in my life, as only having children can be, of course. Over time, it became clear that my son's birth, and that of his sister 10 years later, would have a significant affect on how I would later work with children and their families, particularly as it related to my own experiences as a parent, single parent, and working mother as described below.

After graduating from the occupational therapy program in 1982, I began working for a special education cooperative that served 16 school districts in Chicago's western suburbs. These were primarily affluent, White, middle-to-upper-class communities, and I was the only African American therapist working for the co-op as well as serving the children. For the most part, that wasn't a problem, although there were times when school staff would do a double-take when they saw me coming into the building and I'd have to make sure they knew who I was and why I was there. I did the usual occupational therapy things—conducted evaluations, treated the children, met with teachers, attended individualized education program (IEP) meetings, and documented my interventions. I often had to advocate for what I believed were appropriate services and supports for the students I worked with, even if it meant that occupational therapy would not be provided. At the time, individual disciplines, rather than the full team, usually decided whether a child would get specific services. Many of the teams I participated in rarely had meaningful discussions about what the child really needed to be successful in school. Instead, I was often asked at the beginning of the meeting, "how much OT" I was going to provide over the next year. With IEP meetings scheduled in 15-minute increments, I guess it really was too difficult to have the kinds of necessary conversations to truly understand children's needs and what was the most appropriate way to address them. Besides, the prevailing mindset was that the students were only there to get therapy and the more of it, the better. The problem with that is that when decisions are based on nebulous reasons like "we've always done it this way," or because the parents or another team member wanted services to continue, or "professional judgment," it usually meant the students would get occupational therapy into perpetuity and would rarely be discontinued from services. Even then, I preferred to base my decisions on objective factors—evidence, if you will—such as what had or had not worked for children, what the team wanted the child to be able to do during the school year, and what other supports were in place. (This issue of when a student should or should not receive occupational therapy is one that school-based practitioners and IEP teams continue to struggle with to this day.)

While I was learning the ins and outs of school-based therapy, I was also coming to terms with who I was as a working, single parent. I had to juggle work with taking my son to the doctor, getting him to the babysitter, and making sure he had what he needed. Because I worked, I couldn't always take time off for appointments or parent–teacher conferences (which *always* seemed to be scheduled during my work hours), so I began pushing the various agencies to provide evening or Saturday appointments. If they did not provide them, I would find someone who did.

Later, as my children got older and began going to school, I had to contend with their school's expectations regarding parent involvement, which was usually interpreted to mean volunteering in the classroom, helping to chaperone field trips, and meeting to plan Parent Teacher Association (PTA) events and activities—all during the day. In the districts I initially worked in, this might have been a reasonable expectation because the vast majority of the children had stay-at-home mothers. However, this type of involvement was not possible for me and many other parents in the community I lived in. I couldn't just show up when the school thought I should or to participate in the way the school thought I should. It didn't mean, however, that I didn't care about my children. I found other ways to support their learning and education, such as joining the PTA, making sure homework was done and that they read every day, and ensuring that they got enough to eat and went to bed on time. I also made sure each teacher knew how and when to reach me if something came up at school.

Again, my personal experiences greatly influenced how I worked with families on the basis of their availability, trying to understand their perspectives and working with them where they were instead of where I thought they should be. Because of my experiences as a single mother, I began seeing parents as real partners and made every effort to understand their needs and what was important to them. Never again would I presume to be the I-know-everything-about-all-children-including-yours expert with parents. It was important for me to be respected and for agencies to acknowledge the work I was doing with and for my own children. Now, it was my turn to give it back to the families I worked with.

It was not until I started working on my master's degree that I began to understand the potential for policy and what would later become what I'm calling head-on advocacy—the lobbying with Congress and federal agencies that I would do at the American Occupational Therapy Association (AOTA).

Over the years, I moved from school-based settings to inpatient and outpatient pediatric rehabilitation, early intervention, contract work, home health, other community-based settings in and around the Chicagoland area; I even worked at an Easter Seals facility in downstate Illinois. I worked with affluent families and poor families, White families, Black families, Hispanic families, families who spoke English well, and families for whom English was secondary and who needed an interpreter. I taught CPR, became certified in pediatric neurodevelopmental treatment (NDT), and began copresenting with colleagues on innovative treatments we were doing. Through it all, I was aware of a growing sense of dissatisfaction and frustration with how pediatric occupational therapy services were delivered and with the systems in which I worked. I had always thought of myself as a good therapist and wanted to have a bigger impact than I was. I kept thinking that there had to be a better way to support children and their families, but I didn't know what it was at the time.

So, I went back to school to study child development and family issues in greater depth. Several interesting tidbits about my studies: Aside from the lone physical therapist in some of my classes, I was surrounded by early childhood teachers and administrators who seemed to be primarily interested in learning how to manage a classroom or supervise staff. The PT rarely spoke up in class, so I became the de facto expert on disability by virtue of being the only OT; it was amazing how much practical, real-world information was not part of my master's program curriculum at that time (it has since changed).

Hindsight is always 20/20, but I didn't really care at the time as I was being exposed to something greater than I previously had only tinkered with around the edges. Throughout the 3 years it took to complete my coursework, it became increasingly clear that *policy* was a driving factor in how well the needs of children and their families were or were not addressed in our society and that if we did not truly value and support children and families, how could we expect families to raise their children in the ways we think are important or for children to grow and develop into the kinds of people we wanted them to be? At that time, I only understood policy as the rules and procedures that ultimately govern how children are served by different agencies and programs. Over time, I understood that it was bigger than that. "Ah-ha," I thought, "this policy thing just might be the way I could effect the kinds of changes I wanted to see for kids and their families. But how could I get started?" Enter AOTA.

Advocacy With AOTA

When I came to AOTA in 1993 as the Pediatric Program Manager, I almost immediately began taking advantage of the opportunities presented by our proximity to Washington, DC, and the federal government. I went to meetings hosted by different federal agencies, such as the Department of Education, Health and Human Services, and Department of Defense that were open to the public (there were times when I was the *only* member of the public at these meetings!). I attended coalition meetings with other national organizations, for example, Consortium for Citizens with Disabilities (CCD). I even attended some local government meetings in the District of Columbia and Montgomery County, Maryland, as well. I wanted and needed to know who was who, what they were doing (and saying), and how AOTA and occupational therapy fit into the picture. I was convinced that the best way to accomplish this was to be out of the office getting to know who the players were and making sure AOTA had a seat at the table.

All of this policy work was happening at the same time I was hearing from AOTA members who worked with children. I began to see the intersection between policy and practice. It was critical that I understood their needs and struggles and learned about their successes. Throughout my nearly 13 years at AOTA, members kept me apprised of their issues and challenges and how they dealt with them. This information and these relationships were the foundation for my advocacy efforts on behalf of the association and profession.

As I attended more meetings of various agencies (e.g., the Department of Education, the Department Health and Human Services, the Social Security Administration, the Department of Defense), I learned who the people were and what they did. Over time, I was invited to submit information about occupational therapy or to make comments at the meetings. Because of my growing relationships with the various national organizations, I got to know their staffs, executive directors, and board members. I began spending time with the state directors of special education, school psychologists, early childhood professionals, special educators, researchers, and parent groups at meetings and conferences, and I listened to them talk about what they cared about. And, at every opportunity, I talked about occupational therapy and how AOTA was interested in partnering and collaborating with them. There were some roadblocks, to be sure, but I did not let that stop me from interacting and looking for ways to work together.

Eventually, I began getting invitations to present to this state school administrators conference or that national early childhood technical assistance provider conference. It seems these same national organizations with whom I had interacted wanted to know what AOTA's position was on occupational therapy for children, especially in schools and early intervention settings. I saw these invitations as prime opportunities to spread the word about how occupational therapy can help children, support administrators and programs, and provide ongoing support for practitioners.

Soon I began taking on leadership roles in the CCD, a Washington, DC–based coalition of 100 national organizations advocating for national public policy that ensures the self-determination, independence, empowerment, integration, and inclusion of children and adults with disabilities in all aspects of society. I served as CCD secretary for 5 years and was an active member on several task forces that crafted strategy for dealing with federal policy and regulatory issues related to people with disabilities. I became a cochairperson for the Education Task Force in 2000 and served in that role for 6 years.

Around the time I started cochairing, my role at AOTA also changed. Up to this time, I was based in the Practice Department, and my policy work mostly consisted of meetings with federal agency staff, coalition work, and collaborations with other national organizations on issues related to children and occupational therapy. Although I still did that when I moved into the Federal Affairs Department, now I would also be working directly with members of Congress and their staff. This was a whole new ballgame—one that I was not sure I was ready for.

In many ways, legislative work was not all that different from what I had already been doing: I still had to know the issues, what my message was, and what I was trying to accomplish. That was the easy part. The difference was how, when, and where my message was shared and to whom it was communicated. I had to get to know an entirely new group of people while also learning the federal policymaking system and lobbying process. I had to learn about the different levels of staff, who actually had the responsibility for a given issue within each Congressional office and committee, and who had the authority to do something about it (this was not always the same person), which in turn influenced who I talked to about which issue. I also had to learn the legislative and regulatory processes so that I would know when I had to talk "statutory language," when to talk "report language," and when to talk "regulatory language" (and I thought occupational therapy's vocabulary was convoluted!).

At the end of the day, though, it was all about the relationships I had with members of Congress and their staffs, just as it was in my advocacy with the different agencies, coalitions, and national organizations. Most of the time I worked with congressional staff on our issues. There were some occasions when a Representative or Senator would be directly involved in meetings and discussions or I had the opportunity to meet with them directly (Former Senator Ted Kennedy and his son Representative Patrick Kennedy and Representative George Miller most immediately come to mind). There were even opportunities to work with White House staff on particular issues: Bill Clinton and George W. Bush were in office during my time at AOTA, and I had the privilege of working with both administrations.

One of my most memorable achievements was working on the 2004 amendments to the Individuals with Disabilities Education Act

(IDEA, 2004). I worked with congressional staff and members (Republicans, Democrats, and independents), coalitions, and other national organizations that support children and families and who agree that occupational therapy is a necessary part of that support. It was a challenging 2½ years at times, but we were successful at getting the vast majority of what we wanted in the final bill. The second most memorable achievement was being invited to the White House for the signing ceremony and other events commemorating the 25th anniversary of IDEA in 2000.

Getting Started as an Advocate

Therapists ask me all the time, "How do I get started as an advocate?" Chances are that they're already doing it. Therapists advocate every time they sit down with a team to plan the next steps for a child, meet with a teacher to help him or her modify the environment, listen to a parent express joy about what his or her child can now do, speak at a school board meeting about how budget cuts will affect the quality of educational services, or provide an in-service to early childhood providers on effective ways to include children with disabilities in community-based activities. These are all examples of advocacy in the service of children and families.

Opportunities abound for advocating for children and their families, for the profession, and for AOTA. We have to be open to these opportunities and willing to speak up. We don't need to know the ins and outs of how legislation is created, use fancy language, or know all the details of a particular policy. We just need to talk about occupational therapy; we also need to show it, in the way we work with our clients, and support the profession and our state and national associations, and help decision makers understand why they need us—to "walk the talk."

More than 20 years later, I still remember the school psychologist in a small rural town with whom I had worked as an occupational therapist for 2 years telling me on my last day that although he did not understand occupational therapy any better now than he had when I began working there, he trusted me because over time he had come to see that I really did have each student's best interest in mind. This was a high compliment coming from someone who wielded great power on the team and who had been quite antagonistic toward occupational therapy in the beginning of my work there.

I still remember the grandmother—who was the primary caregiver for a grandson with significant disabilities—of one of "my" kids telling me how much it meant to her to see someone really enjoy being and playing with her child—someone who could accept her grandson for who he was and was not struck by what he couldn't do. Even if all he could do was make facial movements (smile, grimace, frown) and turn toward sounds. That's when I knew I was on the right track.

I still remember seeing with increasing frequency specific references to IDEA posted on the old AOTA School System Special Interest Section (SIS) electronic mailing list (and current SIS forums) from practitioners who understood the importance and role of policy in their everyday work with children and families.

Stories like these mean the most to me. They are indicators that I've been doing something worthwhile, and that is the kind of impact I wanted to have. Although we have some battles ahead, I do believe that AOTA and occupational therapy is very well positioned to leverage the work that we've all done, individually and collectively. That's advocacy. And that's what it means to be an advocate.

References

Dictionary.com Unabridged. (n.d.). Advocate. Retrieved November 05, 2009, from http://dictionary.reference.com/browse/advocate

Individuals With Disabilities Education Act of 2004, Pub. L. 108–446, 20 U.S.C. § 1400 *et seq.*

Merriam-Webster's Dictionary of Law. (n.d.). Advocacy. Retrieved November 05, 2009, from http://dictionary.reference.com/browse/advocacy

Advocacy Resources

AOTA's Legislative Action Center, at www.aota.org

Ounce of Prevention Fund's Early Childhood Advocacy Kit, available at http://advocacy.ounceofprevention.org/site/PageNavigator/ToolsandResources

CHAPTER 32

St. Mary's in a Pneumatic Tube

Diana Steffen Steer, *OT/L*

Excitedly climbing the stairs onto the Frontier Airlines Twin Otter, I couldn't wait to visit St. Mary's, a small, Native Alaskan Yupik village that was a 2-hour flight north of Anchorage, where I live. I was going to provide occupational therapy services to children with special needs. The commercial fishing villages—Unalaska/Dutch Harbor, Cordova, and Dillingham—are multiracial. St. Mary's, however, promised the opportunity to immerse myself in the culture of Alaska's First People, or the Yupik people.

Once on the 20-passenger plane, I peered through the dim light of evening, just barely able to see the other passengers, and wondered where I would sit. Although I was often referred to as petite, I still had to make myself smaller so I could wiggle my way forward between the down-coated shoulders on each side of the pencil-width aisle.

After jamming my bag against the wall of the plane—there was barely enough room for my legs—I sat down and took a deep breath, noting the stale air. My eyes adjusted to the darkness as I watched the flight crew ready the plane for takeoff. Laughing to myself, mostly because no one could have heard me over the sound of the engines, I had the intense feeling I was being flown to St. Mary's in a pneumatic tube, much like the canister used for drive-through banking.

Just as I had watched the lights of Anchorage fade into the distance, I strained my eyes to see through the water-and-grime-stained windows as the lights marking St. Mary's airport came into view. I could see lights from two different locations quite a distance apart and wondered why. Our landing was uneventful and before long, the passengers were in the building amid happy greetings. It was then that I noticed how many passengers had brought bags of food from Burger King or McDonald's on the flight with them. One woman had even brought a birthday cake from Fred Meyers. I waited for my luggage and watched as boxes with TVs, stereo equipment, and DVD players were carried away from the baggage claim area. While planning this trip, it did not occur to me how far from Anchorage I would really be and how much of Alaska is inaccessible by road. Products and services I took for granted would not be available in rural Alaska; they are either barged in by boat when the rivers thaw or transported by plane. Even building materials and modular homes are brought in by barge in late spring.

A woman came up and introduced herself as Kathy, the special education teacher at the elementary school in St. Mary's. Kathy was a rugged-appearing woman, much taller than I. I later learned that Kathy had lived in St. Mary's for 20 years and had shot and skinned her first moose this past hunting season. I threw my bags into the dusty four-wheel-drive Suburban, jumped in, and drove down the gravel road toward the village.

During our 5-mile drive, Kathy graciously answered my many questions as we bumped our way down the road. The airport was at the confluence of the Yukon and Andreafsky Rivers, but the town of St. Mary's was really on the Andresfsky River, which was named after a Russian missionary who had established Russian Orthodox missions along the river. This explained the distance between the clusters of lights I had noted while on the plane. We were going to the elementary school review the students' IEPs, teachers' reasons for referral, and to review the student records as well as set up the supplies I would need for evaluation and treatment and to establish my schedule for the duration of my time with the students.

As we drove along, Kathy tossed out bits of information about my caseload. She was most concerned about a student having difficulty with all aspects of her education and social skills. I thoughtfully considered her words and remembered a student I had developed a life-skills intervention program for with the help of her educational staff. In that situation, the educational staff became more objective through the information I had gathered, such as sensory processing considerations, and could recognize the progress their student had made and could continue to make. Using this information, I could put "tools"—different perspectives or approaches—in the staff's toolbox to use when they needed them. I wondered if Kathy's student might benefit from a similar program.

I knew that in some villages all the buildings were up on stilts, but knowing it and seeing it were two different things. The elementary school was large, gray, and up on huge wood pylons. Kathy pointed out the high school about an eighth of a mile away and the teachers' housing units along the north side of the road. In the light of the next day, I would see that both schools were built similarly, nearly 8 feet off the ground in places, the same height as the newer homes along the ridge of a low hillside. Older houses were on the ground. The stilts provide access to plumbing and wiring, making repairs easier, and provide protection from the seasonal freeze and thaw of the permafrost.

Several four-wheelers and snow machines were parked in front of the elementary school with only a few trucks here and there; I had not seen many roads through town. As Kathy and I lugged my gear up the long flight of metal steps and onto the dusty red floor of the gym, I hoped I had chosen the right assessments to bring. Determining which assessments to bring is always a trick due to differences in students' ages and abilities. It isn't uncommon for me to race around a school searching for rulers, blocks, cards, and other items that would allow me to develop an on-the-spot assessment. Maximizing clinical reasoning and observations as well as related documentation becomes essential. I am continually reaching into my store of basic theories and principles of occupational therapy as well as information from the Sensory Integration and Praxis Test (Ayres, 1989). From this foundation, I can compensate for standardized testing yet develop interventions that are relevant to the student and useful for the staff. Additionally, I have learned to creatively adapt whatever is available into an assessment tool or treatment modality.

As I toured the school, I realized the powdery dust covering nearly everything was dirt, due to the silt-like nature of the tundra soil. Men from the community were playing basketball in the gym, a favorite pastime, but would be done soon. Kathy and I walked into the resource classroom where she worked with the kids during the school day. Then Kathy casually mentioned that I would be sleeping in the elementary school for the night. Cheryl, the speech pathologist, was also here so we would be staying in the school together.

I looked around the room, wondering where the beds were, and became acutely aware of the fact that I would be sleeping on the floor—on someone else's bedding. Then I heard, "Oh, by-the-way the bathroom is down the hall, around the corner, and past the windows on the right—and don't drink the water!" A wave of anxiety washed over me as I began to experience a culture shock that I did not expect. Excusing myself, I retreated down a dark hallway to a deserted office so I could break down in private. I was grateful that through my occupational therapy training I knew methods of self-regulation and breathing techniques to modulate my growing anxiety. I eventually became calm and embraced the challenge. After about 10 minutes and a little food, I called my husband, who was sitting comfortably in our Anchorage home, and he helped me compose myself before returning to work.

Our goodbyes widened the gap between the two different worlds. Despite a night mixed with anxiety and restlessness, I woke up ready for work, eager to get started.

The next day, school started with the familiar rush. I met the student Kathy had talked about the day before. The need for therapeutic intervention was apparent, but support needed to come from consistent expectations; sensory diet including heavy work, such as carrying books to the library or pushing the lunch cart; and opportunities for choices within the academic curriculum. The educational staff seemed relieved to have a new plan they could implement easily, and over time the student's school attendance and compliance improved.

In the classrooms, I worked with students who needed help with their pencil grasp and how they formed their letters. One of my favorite interventions is to make dots on the pencil where the thumb and index finger go, naming each dot after an image of the child's choosing and telling them to make sure their dots don't get away. In their own creative way, teachers had constructed weighted pencils using film canisters filled with buckshot to minimize tremulousness, increase motor control, and proprioceptive feedback.

Other students on my caseload needed to work on core body strength, bilateral organization, and visual–motor integration. One child in particular could not keep his body in the center of his scooter board no matter how hard he tried, but he improved as he practiced pulling himself along a fixed rope.

Another child had difficulty anticipating the trajectory of a bouncing ball and often fell while attempting to catch it. He became more successful when the ball was rolled along the floor toward him in different patterns.

The teacher's assistant was trained how to gradually increase the challenge for each of these children and to build their developmental skills and success. Physical education teachers have a gold mine of gym equipment that can be useful for many occupational therapy activities. Scooter boards, ropes, balls of all sizes, cones, beanbags, and the gym floor can all be used. When time allowed, I taught the teachers techniques known to assist with concentration and attention, such as having the children do push-ups in their chairs and drink water using a straw. Most of the children had an innate curiosity and willingness to try anything that resembled a game.

What the village children needed to learn and the techniques needed to teach it were light-years away from what is generally found in the traditional educational system. Native people living in rural Alaska live a more subsistence way of life, for example, fishing, gathering berries, hunting, preparing and preserving food, and the traditional rituals around these activities. Traditional education is, as we know it, is reading, writing, and arithmetic. These children were very contextual and kinesthetic learners. Being so isolated, the rest of the world could have been another planet. Some of these students would continue with a subsistence way of life, and others would go to college. Unfortunately, some who stayed would enter into a life of addiction. The teachers in this village could only hope that the children gained the skills to access a world beyond them, which perhaps was why I saw so many computers.

One student on my caseload was learning life skills and working at the local courthouse. To help with these skills, his curriculum had been appropriately adapted to include supervised work experiences. He was responsible for sweeping, emptying the trash, filing mail in appropriate folders, and helping organize the environment for various events. He did not seem to have an awareness of time, so that was one of his educational goals. He was more successful with a visual schedule, but used it inconsistently. Initiating a task was also difficult, and supervision was necessary for that reason. The student, his aide, and I walked the quarter mile to the local courthouse—a small, rustic, modular building with all the amenities of a courthouse on the inside in miniature—but with folding chairs instead of benches. Route finding was part of this student's educational curriculum as was working in the courthouse. She was due to graduate, and her curriculum was no longer academic but rather skills for life, and she needed to gain enough independence so she could continue to work in a supported environment.

The student's aide was a Yupik woman named Sarah who was about 55 years old. Sarah was dressed in a *kuspuk*, a hooded, long-sleeved jacket with a wide ruffle around the bottom which is common attire, with a fur parka underneath it and a fur-trimmed hood. As we walked, she shared how as a child her parents had signed a piece of paper, not realizing that she would be taken from her village and raised in an Oklahoma boarding school. Having been raised away from her people, Sarah stated that she did not know their ways very well, but her knowledge of their culture was improving. Over time, I learned that most Alaskan Native families had experienced similar situations. Sarah later enrolled as a student in a distance education program through the University of Alaska. She firmly believed in education and declared that "too many kids are lazy these days and don't want to learn." As I came to know more about Sarah, my compassion for Native Alaskans and the disenfranchised grew and continues to grow as I now work with children diagnosed with fetal alcohol spectrum disorders who also battle anger and frustration at injustices placed on them.

Another day, Cheryl and I walked to one of the two combined hardware and grocery stores in town to get our lunch. There were no cafés open in the winter. Of course, even in summer, one could not be certain about the hours of operation for any of the local merchants. Many people went to fish camp in the summer to build food reserves for winter. Cheryl and I walked through an open field of snow behind the school as we watched a snowmobile with two riders buzz around. We could hear dogs barking in the distance and see an occasional vehicle or person. From our vantage point it felt as though we could see over the edge of the earth in all directions. The river was frozen but visible, and some of the village was positioned on low-lying hills with clumps of trees, patches of snow, and grass dotting the otherwise bare-looking tundra and hillsides.

One of the teachers, who lived in the teachers' housing, had invited us over for dinner and then was going to take us to the Yupik Center to watch the women sewing furs. The Yupik Center is an additional building at the school large enough for the boys to build traditional tools such as fishing weirs to use for salmon fishing in the river and also where the girls could come and learn traditional native skills such as beading and skin sewing—making mittens, parkas, and mukluks (boots) or boots as well as head dresses and baskets. The Yupik Center's purpose is to help the people take pride in their culture and learn the ways of their ancestors.

The housing modules the teachers live in all look the same. When Cheryl and I arrived for dinner and I entered the front door, I nearly walked into a large oil drum and furnace used to heat the two-bedroom efficiency home. Apparently, the homes were built this way so fuel lines would not freeze, nor the fuel be stolen. Our host's name was Ann; she was from the East Coast had come to Alaska to teach at the high school. This was her first year of teaching. We exchanged news about Anchorage and the world in general. She shared about life in St. Mary's: The boys were building fishing weirs to catch fish from the river, and the girls were sewing parkas with furs and making beaded designs in the school's Yupik program. Field trips took on new meaning when Ann shared how she chaperoned a hunting trip in which a bear and a caribou were shot and skinned as part of the learning experience.

Ann walked Cheryl and me to the Yupik Center where we met some of the village girls and their teachers. They were hard at work, quietly laughing with each other and conversing softly. There was no loud or boisterous laughter, and they shyly shared what they were doing. One of the girls was making a headdress and tried it on for all to admire. Others were making mukluks or mittens with beaded designs. When asked where the furs came from, one of the teachers said most were from a fur-trading company in Seattle. One of the younger girls was making a clothespin apron and confidently using a sewing machine. I was inspired by her enthusiasm and tenacity as she learned from her elders. While sewing skins, the women talked about Eskimo dancing the coming Friday and said that we could watch them practice for the regional potlatch—a celebration and remembrance of ancestors and passing on names to the younger children—in the spring. Unfortunately, I would be returning to Anchorage before the spring potlatch arrived.

As we left the Yupik Center and headed for the elementary school "hotel" we passed the playground. Earlier that day I had seen the children playing on the equipment in −20° temperatures with added wind chill. "These kids are tough!" I thought. In Anchorage, the playground is closed and indoor recess is scheduled at 0°.

As we looked up into the night sky, the aurora borealis was dancing in all of her bright and fickle glory surrounded by constellations. Colors of red, green, blue–green, and yellow were dancing and twirling across the sky, much as one could imagine the Yupik women dancing on Friday nights to the music of their traditional songs. Although I was chilled to the bone in the frigid air, I watched the night from the hill where I stood, and it seemed as though I could see into the past. I did not want to move from where I stood. I was dressed in clothing rated to −45°, but I wanted to avoid the risk of frostbite, so reluctantly I walked up the stairs, through the hallways and into the special education classroom. I marveled that my profession as an occupational therapist had given me such amazing opportunities. With my thoughts back to the present, in the warmth of the building, it seemed so incredible that one could cross not only distance, but cultures and move between past and present as well—while flying in a pneumatic tube.

Reference

Ayres, J. A. (1989). *Sensory integration and praxis test.* Los Angeles: Western Psychological Services.

CHAPTER 33

More Than Man's Best Friend

Melissa Winkle, *OTR/L*

When I was 6 years old, my parents surprised me with my very first pet. She was the smallest puppy I had ever seen and cute as a bug. A ball of white fluff and a tail with 10,000 wags. Bug-a-lou was my first best friend and the only being that I truly confided in during my childhood. I had plenty of human playmates and a fairly large family, but they could never offer me what she did. She always listened carefully with a thoughtfully cocked head; never judged; and never, under any circumstances, offered advice. She was always so supportive, just watching and waiting, and she was always prepared to romp in celebration or to snuggle through my defeats.

That said, the meaningfulness of animals in my life is not re-flected by tchotchkes, jewelry, or T-shirts embellished with anthropo-morphic words and illustrations. The human–animal bond is not easily seen and is hard to describe. Some people are born with a connection to animals that others do not understand. For me, it is a peaceful, yet pow-erful, relationship. I refer to it as a *relationship* because for some of us, it is reciprocal. It is a fact that my dogs follow me around the house no matter how many room changes I make. It is a fact that when I am in the early stages of a severe allergic reaction, Melvin, one of my dogs, knows before I do. It is a fact that this chapter will be about how dogs helped create my practice, and none of them cares if they are mentioned in the credits.

The first job I ever had was at a grooming shop. I bathed and brushed dogs for $1 each. I was only 11, so it seemed like a lot of money, and I got to make a lot of new friends. I could always handle the skittish dogs. I grew into new positions, including groomer, pet supply store manager, dog sitter, and veterinary assistant. I was sure that I was des-tined to be a veterinarian until one day a family brought in a young, sick animal that could be treated for $90 or euthanized for $60. I sat on the back steps with the animal in my arms and cried because its destiny was determined by $30. It broke my heart that for whatever reason, the family decision maker could not forecast the potential impact this animal might make in the future for her children and perhaps for her.

I began exploring other career paths and was attracted to the variety of environments that occupational therapists could work in, including with animals.

I learned about assistance dogs from some friends when I was in occupational therapy school. Dogs could be trained to assist individuals with visual, hearing, and physical disabilities. Dogs were actually being trained to work for the same people I was being trained to work for. I also learned that a handful of organizations were placing professionally trained "therapy" or "facility" dogs with health care providers; there were reports that the dogs increased patients' motivation and participation, and some said that even individuals in a coma had increased vital signs in response to dogs visiting.

I somehow convinced the founder of Assistance Dogs of the West to place a fully trained assistance dog with me who could the role of cotherapist for animal-assisted therapy. I promised her I would get assistance dogs covered by third-party pay sources, develop an assessment tool that would help identify good candidates for the use of assistance dogs, and research and measure individuals pre- and postplacement with a dog to justify the use of and payment for assistance dogs as assistive technology options. This was a lot for a student to promise, but she saw my passion, and so it was agreed.

Two days after I graduated from occupational therapy school, I went to the placement training course to learn how to work my assistance dog (service variety). I attended the course with people with disabilities who were also getting dogs, and by the fifth day, I knew I was supposed to develop my occupational therapy practice to include not only animal-assisted therapy but assistance dogs.

Over the past 8 years, I have seen some incredibly fast progress. The motivation and participation of both dogs and clients grew to exceed the resources I had. I was able to develop new intervention strategies so naturally and quickly that I was losing sleep trying to capture it all. And the more activities that were developed, the more progress clients made. My practice took on a life of its own. I have seen children who were on feeding tubes begin eating orally because they developed trust after hand feeding a dog. Others with gravitational insecurity began climbing a course led by a dog. Initial fasteners and shoe tying were more interesting to the kids; handwriting was no longer so stressful when it was used in conjunction with activities with the dog.

Adults with developmental disabilities were enjoying counting money to purchase dog treats and supplies used in sessions. Soon, they were looking at recipes (person- and dog-friendly) to make grocery lists, finding bus routes to stores, shopping, managing money, and following written instructions to make the tasty treats. They were learning sign language to interact with the dog and teaching the dog new skills. They were teaching the dog new skills!

Within a few years, my practice partnered with Assistance Dogs of the West and an adult day program facility to develop a pilot program of intervention services. I did not exhale for the first few months. We had to learn how to teach our new student trainers how to train the dogs. It required eye contact, timing, fine and gross motor skills, communication, problem solving, and so much more! It was a success because the dogs never critiqued them. If a dog does not get a clear message, it will try something it does know, or it will wait for something interesting to happen. The clients did not get easily discouraged because all they had to do was keep trying until the dog understood.

Now, my clients, who had developmental and physical disabilities and traumatic brain injuries, were training assistance dogs for Assistance Dogs of the West, who then placed them with other community members with disabilities. My clients and I went to malls, grocery stores, restaurants, and many other public venues to train dogs. For the first time in many of my clients' lives, their disabilities were seen as a gift. In fact, there was no other way to get into our program at the time. My clients were approached by community members, advocated for themselves and the training of the dogs, and later the people who received the dogs. I could finally exhale!

The skills learned by the students were many, and people were beginning to notice. The crew from the *Today* show came and followed the program participants and then flew a few of us to New York City for a live taping for the segment titled "Today's Heroes." After the show aired, Assistance Dogs of the West was in some magazines and the local newspaper. Our student trainers had superstar status. Peers and case managers asked them to autograph the articles or to stop for photos. They were recognized in the mall!

We soon had to expand our services. Dogwood Therapy Services was born. We developed new animal-related community programs for vocational training and integrated after-school assistance dog training programs and basic obedience dog-training classes where clients could train their own dogs. We began to develop plans for clients to open their own small businesses in animal-related fields, including dog sitters, dog walkers, turtle garden landscapers, and the like.

The animal-related portion of the business has always been the most popular, the most challenging, and the most progress generating. We have watched our clients come into integrated community programs just to work with the animals but walk away with friendships with individuals who may or may not have disabilities.

Dogwood Therapy Services has been recognized by the American Occupational Therapy Association for the emerging practice areas of animal-assisted therapy and interventions and assistance dogs as assistive technology options. We are currently involved in five research projects. We offer continuing education courses on animal-assisted interventions, assistance dogs, and program development. We are working on a book and continuing education DVDs, which will propose higher standards of practice for health care providers using animal-assisted therapy and interventions in practice. We now have people coming for postprofessional continuing education and consultation services from four countries. More than three-quarters of our clientele has been referred to us for programming, which involves animals and integrated services. I remember when I waited to exhale to see if this would all work, now it just takes my breath away. My clients are living life to the fullest, and so am I.

CHAPTER 34

The Challenges and Joys Faced by the Sandwich Generation

Barbara Smith, *MS, OTR/L*

It's a challenge for any caregiver to live life to its fullest. After all, taking care of a person with a disability is not only time consuming and expensive, it's emotionally draining as well, leaving little time for professional and personal pursuits. I had been an occupational therapist for 15 years when I became my mother's caregiver. Fortunately, occupational therapists are equipped with special skills to help loved ones maximize abilities and access services. We also understand how important it is to meet our own needs to achieve balance and self-fulfillment. Occupational therapy practitioners know how to be flexible, creative, and recognize the value of small gains. Although nobody chooses to be thrust into a caregiving situation, once we accept the inevitable, we can pursue the role with vigor and success.

In my situation, I identified my mother's early symptoms of Alzheimer's disease about 10 years ago when she began getting lost while walking in her community, living on crackers and chocolate, and neglecting her hygiene. I had never before worked in geriatrics, except for the occasional older client with developmental disabilities whose increasing senility seemed like a natural progression given his or her lifelong cognitive limitations. Therefore, it was unsettling, to say the least, when my mother was suddenly the one with cognitive needs that would eventually be greater than those of the clients I served.

At this time I was mother to a 10-year-old son who had always been hypersensitive to sensory stimuli, highly distractible, and socially anxious. I never felt a need to label his differences, but eventually obtaining a diagnosis of Asperger's syndrome in high school enabled my husband and me to seek out school accommodations. Ironically, I worked in a school system and performed evaluations, occasionally playing a decision-making role as to what occupational therapy services a child with Asperger's syndrome would receive. The parents were often angry and resistant to any decrease of services after years of therapy to improve handwriting or organizational skills. As a mother of a struggling prepubescent child with my own battles, I had found the school setting stressful. However, working school hours enabled me to be home with my son after each stressful day of academic and social challenges.

Fortunately, I never had to perform the heroics of a primary caregiver, because my mother's financial situation enabled her to live in a beautiful and caring private-pay assisted-living facility. The memory impairment unit provided 12 hours of daily recreation and entertainment. Other people were paid to supervise mom's day-to-day self-care needs while I got to walk with her in the garden or participate in word games, exercise group, or sing-alongs. During the early stages of the disease I looked forward to taking Mom out of the nurturing but regimented day program, and we spent many afternoons dining out, taking in chick flicks, and walking through lovely parks. We developed some fun routines, and mom accepted my interventions when I helped in the bathroom stall, ordered sandwiches when she could no longer manage a fork and spoon, or bundled her up on a snowy day as we made our way to a medical appointment.

As the parent of a child with social challenges, I never got to join the network of soccer moms, nor did I form the friendships that evolved out of shared parenting experiences. However, as I got to know the staff and families of other residents in mom's assisted-living facility, some of my own social needs were met. These were the people who appreciated my mother for who she was at this time in her life. Like most with Alzheimer's disease, my mother lived in the present; past grievances dissolved, the future was unspoken. Her unconditional love and simplicity provided respite from my stress-filled life.

While my mother's mental status gradually deteriorated during her 3 years living in the assisted-living home, my son plodded through middle school. Homework that might take a typical child 2 to 3 hours, took 5 to 6 hours for a child with attention deficit disorder and anxiety, leaving little time for exercise or play. He often woke up during the night with school-related nightmares. As occupational therapy practitioners know, middle school is also a time when adolescents develop more complex social networks, and kids enjoy socializing in groups. This change in social expectations is difficult for people who process language best in a one-on-one situation. My son's childhood friendships based on common interests in camping and building fizzled out when relationships required more complex verbal skills. My mother and son were both struggling to communicate, and I was struggling to listen.

As my mother's disease advanced, I continued to read all the books about Alzheimer's disease, both those written for occupational therapists with adaptation ideas and those written by spouses or adult children that dwelled on the challenges of finding a caring and affordable facility. I read books written by the people with Alzheimer's disease themselves, who used writing to cope, record, and feel useful. Then I read the many medically oriented books touting the latest wonder drugs on the horizon that would dissolve the gooey plaques and tangles in the brain and how to keep our brains young with cod-liver oil and crossword puzzles. What I ultimately learned was that my mother was a very lucky lady to have a daughter who was an occupational therapist.

When Mom could no longer remember to use the toilet, the nurse at the assisted-living facility asked me to move her out. An occupational therapist friend recommended a nearby nursing home that happened to have an available private room overlooking the patio. It seemed too good to be true, and it was. Watching Mom leave her safe, happy home was like seeing my child be expelled from Harvard to attend a poorly funded community college. In the nursing home, organized activities only occurred for 1 hour in the morning and another hour in the afternoon, and they were mostly designed for higher-functioning residents. Mom no longer understood how to play bingo, nor could she follow a discussion.

I put my occupational therapy background to use as I advocated (to no avail) for my mother to have more stimulation and suggested that the recreation staff adapt activities for lower-functioning individuals. Because Mom spent many hours alone in her room, I created activities that she could enjoy independently. Mom obsessively read the illustrated story of her life that I wrote and could be heard belting out the large-print 1940s song lyrics I compiled into a binder. (These and other activities designed for individuals with memory impairment can be viewed on my Web site, BarbaraSmithOccupationalTherapist.com.) Instructions for the staff were hung on the wall so that they would play her Broadway musical CDs instead of parking her front of a television. In addition, I made up word games for the two of us to play when normal conversation was no longer possible.

As a middle-aged sandwich generation daughter, my life increasingly centered on helping my mother and my son. This situation could not be changed. However, I thought finding a more interesting occupational therapy job might improve my mental health. When my son graduated high school I immediately set out to find a work setting where I could learn new skills and excel. Although I had no experience with horses, I decided to get a job working at a hippotherapy facility where horses were used as treatment tools. My young clients arrived happy with anticipation. Nonverbal children could show off their skills to change positions, steer with reins, and sign to go and stop. Parents felt hopeful in knowing that their children not only improved their motor and language skills but also got to ride a horse—an experience many other children could only dream of. When I realized that hippotherapy was the field for me, I took the certification courses and began learning how to ride an animal that often acted like a stubborn 3-year-old.

My son has always loved sensory stimulation. He was never defensive and was in his glory when holding mud, smelling play dough, or sleeping with a big piece of fur. He must have inherited this trait from me, because I also love new sensory experiences. Working with and riding horses provide intense tactile, vestibular, and proprioceptive stimulation—whether brushing their coats, carrying a saddle, trotting, or lying prone while facing the horse's tail. My mother was entering her own sensory stage. She liked to hold objects that were soft, vibrated, or made sounds when moved.

As my mother entered the late stages of Alzheimer's disease, I decided that I wanted to share not only her story and my challenges but also the solutions that often came to me during sleepless nights. Google the word "Alzheimer" and you will find hundreds, if not thousands of books already written on this subject. So why did I want to write another? I have always loved memoirs, and they can make an otherwise dry subject readable, even suspenseful. *Still Giving Kisses: A Guide to Helping and Enjoying the Alzheimer's Victim You Love* (published by lulu.com, 2008) is designed to entertain as well as inform. But foremost, I wrote this book to give caregivers the tools to enjoy the person with Alzheimer's disease. The person may not be able to verbalize how important visitors are, but personal attention is nevertheless critical. Writing and lecturing about my book is also part of a healing process that allows me to continue caregiving even though my mother has passed away.

Today my son attends college, is exploring career options, and getting rather good at self-advocacy. Because I love a challenge, I have joined the public-speaking organization Toastmasters, Inc. to brush up on my presentation skills. I have faced many obstacles as a sandwich generation caregiver but have also had wonderful experiences that I am ready to speak about. To me, living life to its fullest means making the best of a bad situation and then making it even better.

Reference

Smith, B. A. (2008). *Still giving kisses: A guide to helping and enjoying the Alzheimer's victim you love*. Raleigh, NC: Lulu.com

CHAPTER 35

How to Get Your Light On

Marjorie Vogeley, *MGA, OTR/L*

> Note. *This was the presidential address at the 2009 Maryland Occupational Therapy Association's Annual Conference in Timonium, Maryland.*

This year's theme for the Maryland Occupational Therapy Association's (MOTA's) Conference is "Make OT Shine in 2009." Light is so attractive; be it a sunrise or sunset, the lamp in the window at home, the flickering candle on the restaurant table—people are drawn to a light. The year 2010 is around the corner with challenges old and new; I want you to be ready and to shine. So the subject for my address today is "How to Get Your Light On."

I'm not sure when it was that I first had to define *occupational therapy*, but most certainly it occurred when I was an occupational therapy student. Without a doubt, I know that on some quiz or test I had to write the definition of occupational therapy, and it was likely quoted word for word from that year's trusted *Willard & Spackman* textbook. After those many weeks, months, and years of learning, I anticipated that I would be thoroughly educated and knowledgeable about every aspect of the concept of occupational therapy.

Despite all that wonderful instruction, in looking back at my first years of employment, my "green behind the ears" years, I really had no clue. Oh, I knew the concept of occupational therapy, and I could perform the job that I was hired for, but as time went on it became all too obvious that it was one thing to do it—to "provide" occupational therapy—and altogether another thing to actually embody it. That state of being, where you have processed the idea and spirit of occupational therapy so that it comes naturally and easily for you to communicate and share it with another human being—*that's* getting your light on.

The beginning of my career was humbling. My first job was in a spanking new rehabilitation hospital in the middle of Texas. I would tell my patients that I was the one who would help them get back into doing their daily activities like dressing or cooking. I should have guessed that this was not always an effective way of promoting occupational therapy because my patients' retorts sometimes read like the options listed in a multiple-choice question:

1. "What do I need that for? I have a wife for that."
2. "I just need my rest. When I get home, I'll be able to do all of that."
3. "There's nothing wrong with me." (The answer of choice for the people with left-sided hemiplegia)
4. "I don't need occupational therapy. I just need to walk. Take me to physical therapy."

When I couldn't sell my explanation of occupational therapy, I would usually put on my poker face, imagine that I laid my cards on the table, and speak as if I had the upper hand: "Your doctor ordered it, so you will be coming to occupational therapy and working with me."

The process of "getting my light on" truly began one day at that Texas rehabilitation hospital when I entered a patient's room to introduce myself. I vividly recall enthusiastically telling my new client, an elderly man who was gazing at the ceiling and lying supine on his hospital bed, that I was his occupational therapist. To this, his head turned slowly to me, and he rolled his eyes. Then he parted his lips and with a long, southern drawl (or more appropriately, a Texas twang) he said, "Honey, I doh-n't need no job. Can't you tell I'm re-tyr-ed?"

That man left me, for once, at a loss for words. I have never forgotten his very clever comeback. That moment was the beginning of a whole new outlook for me; it began a journey of defining and redefining my ideas and explanation of this concept of occupational therapy.

You've heard my mantra for this association—"Stand Up for Your Profession"—many times. It was this incident in Texas, 30 years ago, which made me realize how important it was to be able to explain to others what I stood for.

Over the span of many subsequent jobs, several evolutions of explaining occupational therapy occurred. Men particularly appreciated my "fewest words answer" which seemed to elicit more cooperation than any other explanation that I could give. I simply stated, "The word *occupational* refers to 'how you are occupied,' so I'm the one who's going to help you get back to doing what you normally do." Function became the emphasis of choice rather than any particular activity. However, periodically my patients would still equate function with the singular task of walking and wanted to steadfastly focus only on that. I wish

I had been as quick-witted as my colleague, Rae Ann Smith, who when faced with the same situation asked her patients just one question: "So you want to walk naked?"

Clients haven't always been bold enough to ask me, "What is the difference between occupational and physical therapy?" which I feel is essential to explain—else you'll never get the full credit for what you do, and your work might be referred to as the "other physical therapy." People define things based on what they see, so I had to speak up when patients reflected that occupational therapy meant working from the waist up. My response to them customarily was "In occupational therapy, we are concerned with how you are occupied. People occupy themselves with activities. An occupational therapy practitioner will use activities in a therapeutic way. And generally, to perform an activity you need the use of your arms and hands. This is why we are particularly knowledgeable and skilled in rehabilitation of the arms and hands, but that's only one aspect of occupational therapy. We address a person's entire functioning."

That was my embodiment of occupational therapy several years ago. I felt I was good at telling others about what occupational therapy represented, but it was slightly flawed because often I explained it through the context of how occupational therapy measured up to other professions.

Working in various skilled-nursing facilities brought to light how I needed to stop focusing on what I was all about. When I first performed my evaluations, I wanted the answers to questions such as these: "How well does this person understand me?" "Can I get this person to roll over?" "Where are the joint limitations and contractures?" "When I ask this person to push, will I get a reliable measure of her arm strength?" "How much help does this individual need from me in putting on her blouse?" At least I can say that I was a better assessor than some other professionals, who would march into the room, straight up to the reclining patient, and then demand that the person pull this, lift that, straighten up, sit up, and stop being so scared to transfer over to the wheelchair.

Many of those same patients later in the week would be sitting in the rehabilitation department, parked at the worktable, chatting idly with whomever would be nearby, and using sophisticated vocabulary in their conversation. And if you listened, truly listened, you were struck that this wasn't a "*patient*" but someone with a wealth of knowledge. This was a "*person*," one who had a story to tell.

I was getting my light on. The first thing of importance wasn't to get this measurement or that test done. What was important was listening to the story and learning about that person. How could I be an effective occupational therapist without understanding what it was that this person wanted and desired, even if it was to be left alone? What had their life been like, yesterday, last week, last year, 20 years ago? What were this person's resources? But more than that, this never was about what I could provide, but rather, how I could be a vehicle for this individual and infuse occupational therapy concepts into her being, so that she could reengage in function and be effective in her own right returning to and performing activities that were meaningful and important to her. I had come face-to-face with the concept of "therapeutic use of self."

For the past 2 decades, I have had to apply that thinking to a different context as an occupational therapist employed by a school system. Where I once focused on addressing the child's disability at school, I now focus on the barriers and supports that permit the child to access, participate, and progress in his or her educational program. The school-based therapists who have their lights on know that merely possessing a disability does not matter at school. What is important is this—by virtue of a disability, one can't obtain an education. And I use that word in the broadest sense, for school systems are slowly acknowledging that obtaining an education doesn't exclusively mean the three Rs of reading, writing, and arithmetic: general education curriculum should contain supplemental indicators of learning and achievement, such as a student's level of interactional skill development to complete a group project in class or organizational skills so that work content can be delivered on time and intact to be graded. School-based therapists who know what they stand for never have to ask the question, "Does this student need occupational therapy to implement his or her IEP?" The writing on the wall is clear. The only decision that needs to be made is which avenue is best: direct or indirect?

My education broadened this year after several visits to the Maryland General Assembly. The athletic trainer's licensure bill went before the Maryland House of Representatives and Senate. Our MOTA lobbyist and I visited various delegates and senators prior to this bill being heard in the respective committees. The very first legislator we visited was cosponsoring the athletic trainer's bill in the House; that meant of course, this politician had a vested interest in this bill passing.

I wanted to have my light on, but the "glow" I felt wasn't coming from within. What initially started as a pleasant meeting, turned out to be a grilling with me as the main course over the hot coals. The legislator made it clearly understood that he would not tolerate "turf wars" over services; athletic trainers were recognized as health professionals, and they were qualified to treat injuries. He pointedly told me that the consumer should be able to get treatment from his or her provider of choice.

A few weeks after that visit, I provided testimony on the athletic trainer's bill to the Maryland Senate Education, Health, and Environmental Affairs Committee. On that day, all those years of defining and redefining occupational therapy as I knew it, my long road engaging and practicing the art and science of occupational therapy—all of it— came to a crowning moment. I discussed the need to define in the bill who qualified as an athlete, which was a point of contention surrounding the topic of scope of practice with the professional groups. I sat at the microphone and told the Senate committee that I felt it was important for athletic trainers to only address "athletic injuries." I recalled a previous conversation I had had with the president of the Maryland Athletic Trainers' Association. I had disagreed with the president, who adamantly informed me that the athletic trainer's services should not be limited to just athletics: "An athletic trainer is qualified to treat an ankle injury whether it's on the field or off. An ankle injury is an ankle injury, you follow the same protocol."

Then I sat upright and looked at the panel. It was time to tell the committee and athletic trainers not only what I stood for, but to lay it on the line. "The athletic trainers, they think all injuries are the same. This is exactly why their practice must be limited to athletic injuries. Let me tell you the important difference between athletic trainers and occupational therapists. I don't treat injuries. I treat *people*—and they are *not* all the same."

The room suddenly hushed, and I felt a bit warm. With that, I knew I had got my light on.

Index

About the Editors

Ashley M. Hofmann is the Development/Production Editor for AOTA Press at the American Occupational Therapy Association; she previously was a staff writer for *OT Practice*. She graduated from Occidental College in Los Angeles, California, with a degree in women's studies and a minor in English, and earned her master's degree in English from the University of Virginia.

Molly V. Strzelecki is the Senior Editor for *OT Practice* at the American Occupational Therapy Association. She graduated from Saint Mary's College in South Bend, Indiana, with a degree in creative writing. Her work has also appeared in the *Baltimore Sun* online and DC Metromix online.